BEYOND AIDS

A Journey Into Healing

DEDICATION

This book is lovingly dedicated to all those facing a fatal diagnosis and who have been given a death sentence by those whom they have turned to for help. Through sharing our search for inner peace and healing it is my hope and prayer this book will become one more candle shining in the darkness, lighting the path for those who seek the incredible love and power that exist within them. Whether this journey culminates in a physical healing of the body or a healing into death, it is not the destination, but in each step of the path that the real healing is experienced.

BEYOND AIDS

A Journey Into Healing

George R. Melton
in collaboration with Wil Garcia

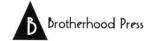 Brotherhood Press

Copyright © 1988 by George R. Melton
All rights reserved.

ISBN: 0-9621959-0-1

No part of this book may be reproduced or utilized in any
form or by any means, electronic or mechanical,
including photocopying, recording, or by any
information storage and retrieval system, without
permission in writing from the publisher.

Brotherhood Press
279 South Beverly Drive, Suite 185
Beverly Hills, CA 90212

First Printing 1988
Second Printing 1989

Cover design by Ron Scarselli
Book design and composition by
Leena Hannonen, Macnetic Design
and Charlie Swanson
Cover photo by Jack Lardomita

First edition 1988
Manufactured in the United States of America

ACKNOWLEDGMENTS

First and foremost, I would like to acknowledge Wil Garcia. This book is as much his as it is mine. Without his love and support, I would not have had the will to make this journey alone. In addition, it was his willingness to transcribe my long hand text onto the word processor that allowed this project to be completed in a reasonable amount of time. For all this and more, I am grateful.

I would like to acknowledge my many teachers. The work of Edgar Cayce has had a profound effect on my understanding of Christianity and my relationship to God. The many books of Jane Roberts and Seth played a major role in teaching me about the power of my own mind. I am grateful to the beautiful work of Sanaya Roman and Orin for its power and simplicity. I would also like to thank Louise Hay.

I would especially like to acknowledge Mark Victor Veneglia for his incredible talent and vision. Without his encouragement, I might never have come forward to tell my story. I would also like to thank Charlie Swanson for his efforts on my behalf in bringing this book to life. Special thanks to Gregory Flood for his many suggestions. I would also like to thank Eric Bailes, Barry Becker, Henry DeNome, Dana Faber, Douglas Grey, Leena Hannonen, Christopher Macklin, Ken Melton, BettyClare Moffatt, Laura Norvig, Patrick, the Power Seven, Leslie Roberts, Mark Rogers, Ron Scarselli, Bill Sullivan, and my entire clientele for their love and support.

I am grateful to the living presence of God within for the unwavering love and wisdom that has brought me through this far.

CONTENTS

PREFACE

In the beginning we were told that everyone who contracts the dread dis-ease AIDS would die and most of them in less than one year. I have never accepted this blanket verdict. I have always known that no experience, no matter how intense, is fatal to everyone. Individuals survive earthquakes, fires, bombings, holocausts, plagues, plane crashes, and dis-eases like cancer. Surely AIDS could not be different.

Now, as time passes I am discovering more and more people who are indeed healing themselves from the dis-ease called AIDS. They have decided to become part of their own healing team and to go beyond all so-called limitations placed upon them by others.

George Melton and Wil Garcia are two such people. They are wonderful examples of what can be done when we go within ourselves to find the extraordinary capabilities we all have. When we believe in ourselves and the powers within us, then we can astound others with our accomplishments.

George, in telling their story, brings hope to those who have been in despair. He shares with us their experience in healing. In doing this he opens endless possibilities for those who wish to explore their own abilities in their healing process.

I truly believe that we can rise above all obstacles if we are willing to explore and discover our own healing powers within us. I encourage you to read this book and join the ranks of those who have moved through the valley of the shadow of death and to walk in the sunshine of life once again.

Louise L. Hay
Santa Monica, CA
September, 1988

FORWORD

For too long, media reports have presented sensational and distorted stories about AIDS. For too long, the prophets of doom have held sway among us. It is now time for the truth to be told and for hope to be reclaimed. Contrary to what we are being told, hundreds, if not thousands, of individuals are thriving—not necessarily because of modern medical science, but in spite of it. These "survivors" have discovered their way out of the darkness.

This book is the dramatic record of two courageous individuals. George Melton's clear and powerful message will stand for all times as an example of things possible for those who are willing to take charge of their own lives. It is a testament to the power of a focused human mind which is willing to change.

Scientists now understand that the brain is a giant immune gland, which is turned on by love, hope, and joy. This command control center is turned off by fear, depression, and anger. Can anyone argue that American medical establishment, with the complicity of the media, has not woefully fostered fear and depression in the immune systems of broad segments of the American public? In truth, no epidemic has ever been 100% fatal, even among those who develop symptoms.

There are many explanations why we are beginning to see long-term survivors. It is my opinion that the true cause of AIDS is not the relatively weak HIV, virus but comprehensive immune system weakness occurring as the result of a modern lifestyle which includes prescription and illicit drugs, poor nutrition, promiscuity, negative attitudes, and an impoverished spiritual nature. With a shift in attitude, proper nutrition, and focused spiritual concerns, a person's revitalized immune system can abolish the milieu which fosters opportunistic infections, including HIV. The AIDS viruses can be contained and put back to sleep just like all the other germs which are continually entering our bodies naturally.

Persons with AIDS must make every effort to seek out survivors and their stories and to model their successes. The way to success is not easy, as the author demonstrates. Anyone with AIDS or who is worried about it will find this book especially valuable. George and Wil's story vividly describes the patterns of intense searching and discovery which I have observed on other long term survivors, and about whom I reported in my books *Healing Aids Naturally* and *Choose To Live*.

Survivorship is a total effort. Aspirant survivors must seek out their own custom-made programs. With persistent searching, it is possible to discover the key, unchanging principles of nature. The application of these principles in a natural healing program will differ from person to person. No two survivors will evolve exactly the same program of nutrition, exercise, attitudinal shift or spiritual focus.

You will learn dramatically in BEYOND AIDS that a critical part of any survivor's healing program are attitudinal shifts and development of a firm sense of self-worth and self-esteem. Love of self is critical for potent functioning of the immune system, the body's system of self-preservation. When people love themselves, their body's servomechanisms turn full speed ahead toward constructive operation. When mental feedback to the unconscious mind contains images of low self-esteem, the unconscious mind "gets the message" and causes the immune system to switch to a destructive mode. The result is AIDS.

Aspiring survivors, go out and take charge of your life, and as you do so you will take charge of your immune system. At the very moment you decide to take control, your healing will begin. Generate a new reality. Avoid those who would disempower you in your search for healing. Follow George Melton and Wil Garcia's bright light into the realm where Body, Mind and Spirit are all One. As you follow in their footsteps, always remember that your Self is the only One who can make it happen.

Laurence E. Badgley, M.D.
Natural Therapies Medical Group
Santa Monica, CA
September, 1988

INTRODUCTION

Only a little more than five hundred years ago the world was flat. Each morning the sun rose in the east and set again in the west at the end of the day. Everyone believed this was true. It was obvious to the eye. In fact, these beliefs had not only the full backing of the scientific community at that time, but the seal of approval from God, via his spokesman on earth, the clergy.

At that time, Europe had become a crowded and troubled place. In spite of this, no attempt to sail away in search of undiscovered lands was even dreamed of. It was not within the realm of possibility on an earth that was flat. Everyone was afraid even to wade too far from shore, for alas, one could see with his own eyes, things drifting out to sea eventually fell off the edge. Everyone knew this was true.

Everyone, that is, except one very clever fellow. Through studying the sky and the movement of the stars, he came to the startling conclusion the world was round. Unfortunately for him, upon reporting his findings to the public he was declared a lunatic. He was even excommunicated by the church.

Eventually however, a few brave people began to suspect what he had said just might be correct. They began to ponder the implications of living on a world that was round. Finally a few of these brave men took to the sea in ships, willing to face the unknown in search of the truth.

These men proved the world was round. They also discovered the sun really never rises or sets. They explored new lands and met exotic people. The entire face of the earth was transformed by this new awareness.

The truth is the earth was never flat. It was always round. The only thing that changed back then was man's understanding of it. As they changed their minds, they changed their experience.

Now, hundreds of years later, we are faced with an epidemic of AIDS. It is believed by almost everyone to be incurable. The full integrity of the scientific community stands behind the complete fatality of this disease. Many of our religious institutions believe it is divine retribution from God. And those few doctors and clergy who have had the intelligence and integrity to stand forth and question these assumptions have been denounced as quacks and ridiculed unmercifully.

Now, as many years ago, a few brave men and women have begun to ponder the possibility that AIDS can be healed. And many of them have set sail on their own journeys of discovery, seeking against all odds to find the truth. Now, from different quarters, we have begun to hear of people who are long term survivors, people who have recovered from AIDS. We don't hear too much, however, because no one wants to risk censure. No one wants to give false hope. They feel safer with false fear.

The truth is all disease can be healed. Once again, we stand at a point in time where the official belief systems no longer fit the personal reality. Again, nothing in reality has changed. There has always been a cure for AIDS. The only thing that has changed is some people have allowed themselves to look for the answers where they truly exist, not just where society believes they are.

In the case of a disease such as AIDS, the official medical verdict as a totally incurable disease has completely robbed the infected of hope, seeing them as helpless victims facing imminent death. Without hope, there is no possibility of recovery.

If there is to be recovery, it will be necessary to look beyond the current offerings of the medical profession, toward other areas in which solutions may possibly lie. These solutions lie within the expanded awareness of man as a multidimensional being, far greater than his physical body.

All of the events of life, including wellness and illness, exist as multidimensional experiences. They take place not only on the outer physical surface of our life, but in the interior of our being, within the realms of the mind and spirit. Without a wholistic understanding of the totality that is man, we have no hope of a cure for AIDS. To deal with it effectively, we must address not only the issues of the body, but those of the mind and spirit as well.

The best efforts of our medical sciences have been doomed to failure. Their attempts to treat this disease by fighting its outer manifestations have been to no avail. Like cancer before it, the billions of dollars poured into research will not bring us a cure. It has not been possible to find the solution for this disease within the current western medical paradigm.

For too long, western medicine has been a one dimensional approach to a multidimensional problem. The solution to AIDS will not be found by excluding two thirds of the equation. It will come only from a totally integrated approach involving body, mind, and spirit. Our current fixation with suppressing symptoms has only created bigger symptoms. We need to understand the cause.

The medical hierarchy has too ingratiated itself to the concerns of the major pharmaceutical companies to allow an expanded search for solutions. There is too much pride and money invested in faulty assumptions to truly move forward. If an answer is to be found, it will have to come from other sources.

AIDS has been an incredible challenge to the gay community. In terms of basic self identity and lifestyle, this community has responded with overwhelmingly positive change to the reality of this disease. It has, at last, become a community in every best sense of the word.

So too does AIDS represent as great a challenge to our medical belief systems. It has put the abilities of science to perhaps its greatest challenge. If solutions are to be found, medicine too will be forced into a greater understanding of the very nature of disease. And if it refuses to meet this challenge, it will be a testimony only to its inability to change. Without fundamental change, all of us are left sitting on the dust heap of history, as those with the willingness to embrace new solutions march onward.

The truth is within the reach of every person on this planet. From the truth has sprung every major religion and philosophy the world has ever known. We must look beyond our dated beliefs to the assumptions from which they spring. It is in truth that the healing of AIDS lies. It lies in the knowledge of our true identity and our relationship to the universe in which we live.

Inherent within each problem is the solution to that problem. Within each one of us is a place beyond perception where all knowledge lies. It is here each one of us can go to find the answers we seek. And it is here we can find our vision of a way home. Only then will we even know what the questions truly are.

Many people have trusted their healing to medical science and have died. Many have pursued wholistic and spiritual approaches and died as well. But death, of itself, is not a failure. If that were true, each person on this planet would be ultimately doomed to failure.

For me the issue has become one of life and its quality. To live one day totally free can be more worthwhile than to exist indefinitely under the fear of AIDS. In facing death we can achieve the inner peace and grace that will allow us to know it is but a doorway into another life. Living fully in each present moment is the real issue.

The first section of this book is the story of a search for healing by Wil Garcia and myself. We hope our ideas and experiences will provide inspiration to persons dealing with this disease. It chronicles our search for solutions, from the time of our diagnosis with ARC and AIDS, respectively, until the present time. For us, the search became an exciting journey of self discovery, one in which we were forced to examine our self perceptions at the most basic level. From this examination emerged a new vision of self and purpose for life.

The second section of the book contains the expanded perceptions and understandings of life I awakened to and then acted upon in my healing path. These truths came to me not only in the form of many books and teachers, but directly as inspiration that seemed to come from 'out of the blue'.

While writing these chapters, at times I was aware of being lifted above and beyond my normal perspective to an expanded realm of awareness. I could feel entire blocks of information existing in my mind as if fully completed. As I would write these down, the words would flow effortlessly onto the paper.

Sometimes I would know in advance what was to be written. At other times I would think I was to write about one thing, only to find I had written other ideas I had never been aware of before. These chapters are presented almost identically as they were received.

Beyond AIDS, the creative processes involved in the writing of this book have given me renewed respect for the abilities of our minds and grateful appreciation and awe for the loving presence and guidance available from within.

George Melton

PART I

Our Story

IN THE BEGINNING

AIDS first came into my conscious awareness early in the 1980's by way of various mentions of the syndrome in the gay press. At that time AIDS was making its appearance in only a few isolated cases. Seemingly healthy gay men in the prime of their youth were being struck by this mysterious and as yet undefined malady. It was marked by the appearance of a rare skin cancer. It was usually found in older men of Mediterranean descent. In other cases it was not usually fatal. In these young men, however, it was unusually virulent, attacking the internal organs and leading to death. In many of the cases there was found to be heavy use of 'recreational drugs' and an unusually high number of sexual partners.

I remember making a mental note of these first public notices about this disease but I did not as yet relate it as a danger to myself. Although I was a moderate user of recreational drugs, which sometimes led me to bed with other than my long-time lover, Wil Garcia, I did not consider myself to have a real drug problem. I could not relate to the statistics about the number of sexual partners involved in these cases. After all, I was successfully involved in a full time career and had been living with my lover in a relationship I had enjoyed for over four years.

This was for us both however, the time of the height of our involvement with drugs and the New York disco scene. We were caught up in an endless party that seemed as if it would go on forever. Little did we know how soon it all would come to an end.

My first exposure to a person with AIDS came through my work environment. I was working as a haircolorist in perhaps the largest salon in NYC, employing over seventy people. We operated under a type of "Star System". Those with the greatest client draw and ability to generate a cash flow were more or less able to make their own rules and call their own shots. I had been there for a few years and was in a position where I was practically working for myself. In terms of this "star system", however, there was one haircutter who was literally the top dog in income and the level of celebrity of his clientele. He was an incredibly handsome man in his late 30's with a great deal of creativity and showmanship.

He had swarthy good looks which he highlighted by wearing black leather, giving himself a slightly menacing sexual appeal. His work station encompassed three chairs at the entrance to the salon cutting floor. It was impossible to enter the salon without noticing this man. He had not one, but two assistants who were constantly at his every beck and call. His flare for dramatic presentation made the performance of his work the prime energy generating the overall atmosphere for the entire salon.

His clients would literally wait hours for him to do their hair and this was exactly as he liked it. I heard him say on more than one occasion that he could not work without people waiting and watching. If anyone complained about how long they had to wait, he would tell them to go elsewhere if they didn't like it. He would berate his assistants in front of the clients for the slightest infraction of his rules. In general he was quite arrogant, considering himself to be superior to just about everyone else in the salon.

Even though almost everyone in the shop considered his behavior and treatment of others to be obnoxious, at the same time there was also a strong feeling of admiration and awe for his abilities to get away with this type of behavior. If we didn't particularly like him, we didn't let him know it.

This man was the first person I knew who contracted AIDS. At first he complained of not feeling his energy was up to par and he made innumerable trips to the doctor. No one was able to pinpoint precisely what the problem was. Gradually his condition became more acute. Within a year, he was beginning to take more and more time away from work. Everyone was beginning to notice his conspicuous absences. Rumors circulated he had AIDS, yet he continued to deny it was so.

By this time more information was beginning to be made public about this new disease. Awareness of it as a potential health problem was beginning to grow, as was the increasing fear about possible exposure. After some time this man finally came down with one of the major opportunistic diseases associated with the AIDS condition. He was forced to reveal he did indeed have AIDS. After a long absence, he once again returned to work and the seriousness of his condition was obvious by his physical appearance. He had lost a tremendous amount of weight and his hair was gone due to the radiation treatments he had received for his Kaposi Sarcoma lesions.

With his health steadily failing, he was no longer able to maintain his previous work load. Slowly he was forced to cut back his working hours. One by one his clients began to make arrangements to have their hair done by other people. They left due in part to their own fear and inability to deal with his imminent death.

No longer did he have the dynamic energy so character- istic of his work before the illness. In addition he began to suffer from slight dementia. As his body and life slowly withered away, he would dejectedly walk around the salon in his slack time and talk in the most intimate ways to us about himself, his illness, and his approaching death. In dying, he began to reach out desperately to others in the shop. This was something he had never previously done.

The effect of this on everyone in the salon was devastating. To see a most dynamic man slowly deteriorate into this pitiful figure before our very eyes, was very hard on the morale of the entire shop. No one knew just what to say to him, never having dealt with death in this intimate way before. Everyone began to dread seeing him at work and began as much as possible to discreetly avoid him.

Finally, he could no longer continue to work at all. He returned to his home town and family to await death. If AIDS had seemed to us like a far off thing before, then it's impact had now begun to be felt in a much more personal way.

As time passed, public awareness of AIDS began to grow. Those small articles tucked away in the back of the newspaper began to increase in size and frequency and were moved into prominence on the front pages. And yet it was still labeled just a gay disease. Society as a whole failed to recognize the imminent threat to itself. Instead, people began to make terrible judgments concerning those who contracted the disease. There was still a pervasive sense of denial that AIDS was relevant to "mainstream" life.

As the extent of the crisis continued to grow, insurance companies began to discuss red-lining gay men. The religious right smugly saw it as divine justice, while our political leaders began to ponder such diverse solutions as tattooing and quarantine. In my own personal life AIDS became like an approaching thunderstorm whose lightning bolts could be seen from a great distance. But quickly it began to engulf me, to strike in ever increasing proximity to my personal world.

It began to strike first distant acquaintances who I hardly knew, then friends of friends, and finally friends of my own. It moved ever closer until finally it began to strike at me in a most personal way through those with whom I had been sexually intimate. No longer was it something happening out there to other people. Suddenly the danger was up front and immediate. I had to deal not only with my increasing grief and growing sense of loss at the premature death all around me, but with the now pervasive fear starting to clutch at my heart and lodge in my throat. I could no longer deny I was involved with this disease in the most personal way. There was no doubt of my exposure to the virus.

As the evidence began to pile in from all sides about the correlation between drug abuse, multiple sexual partners, and the contraction of this disease, Wil and I began to slowly extract ourselves from the lifestyle in which we had participated for so long.

Our weekly Saturday night dancing marathons began to occur with less frequency. In our psyche, those evenings were so interwoven with our abuse of drugs that cutting down on one automatically meant cutting down on the other. It meant our opportunities for sexual experiences outside of our relationship, growing out of this drug usage, began to diminish also.

For us it was a very difficult time of change. All of the habitual, unquestioned, behavior of the previous years was being called into question. It now seemed there was a terrible price to pay for the party. Many of our friends continued with the old lifestyle, unwilling or unable to face the imminent changes soon to occur throughout the gay community and then ripple out into the heterosexual world. They were not yet ready to deal with this new reality.

The drugs and music continued to call to us, but we persevered in our determination to make the changes we felt were vital to our very survival. The struggle to break our addiction to drugs was a difficult and painful process. We had not been aware from the surface of things how deep our dependence was. We truly desired to let them go knowing the consequence of not doing so. The habits of many years were in constant opposition to our efforts, however. We began a slow process of finding new activities to fill the void that the loss of these things had created in our lives.

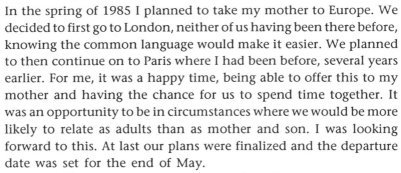

THE LONG SUMMER

In the spring of 1985 I planned to take my mother to Europe. We decided to first go to London, neither of us having been there before, knowing the common language would make it easier. We planned to then continue on to Paris where I had been before, several years earlier. For me, it was a happy time, being able to offer this to my mother and having the chance for us to spend time together. It was an opportunity to be in circumstances where we would be more likely to relate as adults than as mother and son. I was looking forward to this. At last our plans were finalized and the departure date was set for the end of May.

A few days before we were to leave for Europe a very strange rash appeared on my lover's back and right side. Upon visiting the doctor, he was informed he had a case of shingles. Shingles is caused by the chicken pox virus. It lies dormant in the nervous system and if it is triggered into activity in adults, it appears as shingles. The disorder is characterized by a mass of blisters starting from the spine and circling around half of the body to the front, following the path of the affected nerves.

The standard treatment is oral medication and rest, with frequent topical applications of calamine lotion. In almost all cases there is a good deal of pain involved. Wil followed the instructions in treating the symptoms and since there seemed to be no serious danger, when the date of my departure arrived, my mother and I boarded a plane and flew off for our European adventure together.

In London we met up with a cousin of mine and her husband, and we saw the sights of the city together. Upon their leaving London for a tour of the English country side, my mother and I flew on to Paris for the remainder of our visit. The time away together flew by quickly and soon we were back in New York. I waved good-bye as I put Mom on a plane to take her back home to Florida. I hopped in a cab and headed for home. Unknowingly, I was returning to a life that would in no way resemble the one I had left behind. I was about to embark on a totally new phase of my life, one that would leave me forever changed.

While I was away in Europe, Wil made subsequent visits to his doctor in relation to his shingles condition. The doctor informed him that in gay men there was a high correlation between the instances of shingles due to immune damage and the development of AIDS and its related disorders. Studies had shown shingles could be used as a marker for damage to the immune system. Its appearance in an otherwise healthy young man could possibly indicate the onset of AIDS. He suggested Wil have a series of tests performed and various profiles run on his blood in order to better determine the situation.

Being a good patient, Wil consented to have the tests. When the results came back, they were quite startling. His blood profiles showed a dangerously depressed T-cell ratio and the actual number of these cells was very low. On the basis of this and several previous and current conditions, he was diagnosed by his doctor as having ARC (AIDS Related Complex). At a time when I was away on vacation, he was left alone to face and deal with a diagnosis of this severity.

Being the type of person who felt it was his responsibility to live others' lives for them, Wil decided I would be unable to deal with his diagnosis. He felt it would be necessary for him to spare me the experience, one he was sure I could not handle. It was only natural he would decide not to share his diagnosis with me. Being unable to confide in me, he turned instead to his closest friend, Eric Bailes. After telling him the grim news, Eric was sworn to secrecy.

It was to this scenario I returned from the airport, unaware of what had transpired in my absence. They were unable to keep their secret for very long, however. Eric felt it was important they share the diagnosis with me. Reluctantly Wil told me the bad news and then I too was sworn to secrecy. It now became important to both of us that no one know the truth. We had tremendous fear of the consequences if Wil's illness became known.

The weeks that followed dragged on very slowly. We spent weekends in seclusion at our home on Fire Island. We no longer made appearances at the weekend tea dances and our nights partying were no more. Our friends began to see less and less of us as we withdrew into ourselves in an effort to deal with the crisis. Wil was extremely quiet and pensive. I could see he was depressed and afraid of what he feared was to come. Yet he continued to hold his anguish within, as if doing so would protect me from what he believed was the inevitable outcome. We did talk about his condition in a superficial way, but mostly we talked around what we feared the most. It seemed as if there were an invisible wall between us, preventing us from sharing our deepest fear.

The summer passed without any new major physical challenges to our health, but it was definitely not a summer without challenge of an emotional nature. The storm that is AIDS was on top of us now with its full fury, striking all around us at those we loved.

In July, a friend of ours, Larry, went to San Francisco on holiday to celebrate the 4th of July. While he was away, he developed a cough. His friends sent him to their doctor to check out the symptoms. He was immediately hospitalized with pneumocystis pneumonia and began to lapse in and out of coma. Within two weeks he was dead. His death was like a bombshell! Most of his friends had not even known he was sick. Only later did we find out he had known of his condition for over a year. He had chosen to keep his diagnosis secret to himself. He too had been unable to share the burden of his condition with even his closest friends.

How well Wil and I understood the fear that caused us all to keep this deadly secret. The overwhelming fear of rejection and loss was just one more strain on bodies already strained to the limit of survivability. We withdrew inwardly, seeking shelter from the storm.

On the heels of Larry's death, less than one week later, came the death of Wil's uncle from AIDS. He was in his early 50's, a gay man before the generation of sexual liberation. He had never been able to be completely honest about himself with his Hispanic Catholic family. For this reason he had lived a double life with them for his entire life. It was not that they didn't know he was gay, but neither side could bring themselves to broach the subject. As a result, the invisible wall existing within so many gay families had grown up between them, keeping their lives apart. With his death, the family was faced with the loss of a beloved brother without ever having made an effort to remove the wall standing between them. It was not any one person's fault, rather it was a joint conspiracy of silence.

Wil and I attended the funeral together, along with five of his cousins who were gay. It turned out to be a most incredible time of reconciliation. The deceased's lover arranged the service and was there to welcome the bereaved relatives to the service. In death, the family was able to accept the relationship they had not shared with him in life. The recognition of the pain his double life had caused both sides became a catalyst in dissolving those same walls for the others at the service that day. The family was being united in an amazing way.

Knowing the health challenge we faced, Wil was determined what had been true for his Uncle's life would not be allowed to repeat itself in his own life. He could see more clearly now, by the example of his uncle's life, how the secrets he was keeping were barriers between him and those he loved. Several weeks later, Wil made a trip to visit his father. Inspite of his fears of rejection, he told him all the things about himself he had hidden for so long. He was not yet ready to share his illness however. The painful wound of his uncle's death was still too fresh. Instead, he talked about our relationship, his hopes, his dreams. His father, still feeling the pain

of his brother's death, responded by accepting him that day for who
he really was. A long festering wound had begun to heal.

    And so the summer came to a close. It had been a summer
of personal crisis and yet it had its share of triumphs also. I was
at last being accepted by Wil's family. The entire coloring of both
of our lives had been dramatically altered. We had been forced to
face issues of life and death which most people don't encounter
until old age. The death toll of our personal friends and acquaintances was steadily mounting and now Wil was facing his own
mortality. For myself, I was somewhere between facing these issues
as they related to me, and half denying this was my problem at
all. In my mind I had played through many different scenarios of
what the future might hold but always at a distance, always an an
observer separate from the action. I had considered the impact Wil's
death would hold for me, the fear and pain of that being very real.
And yet I never considered the issue of my own mortality. It was
always in terms of the impact Wil's death would hold for me, how
I would survive the pain of the loss. I refused to consider the
implications of being the lover of an infected person, that I too
was probably harboring the same virus. In my mind I had already
disposed of the entire situation and was ready to continue on with
my life as I had in the past. These denials were soon to be faced
head on.

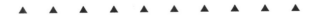

    In early September, our doctor suggested it might be a good
idea for me to submit to a few blood tests. His reasoning was that
since Wil was my lover of many years, there was a high probability
that I had been exposed to the virus. In terms of my previous sexual
history, I knew I faced exposure from many sources. Although I
was generally feeling well, I was suffering from chronic swollen
glands and occasional night sweats. I was worried about these

symptoms and so agreed to have the tests.

My main reason for agreeing was to secure medical confirmation that my health was OK. I wanted proof that this crisis was not my own, that I could take my personal life off hold as it had been for the previous six months. In my mind I reasoned that even though Wil might be facing death and I would be there to support him through whatever happened, there was no reason why my life could not continue on.

The test results were to change all that. My blood profile was nearly identical to Wil's. In fact it was slightly lower for some tests. My T-cell count was severely depressed and my gammaglobulin levels indicated my body was fighting a severe infection.

The effect of these test results were devastating for me! No longer could I hold myself apart from what was happening to Wil. No longer was it a question of what would happen to me after his death. It was now a question of my own survival. I could no longer deny my mortality. The lightning bolt of AIDS had finally struck home!

I didn't know it then, but I realize now as I look back that this was where my healing began. It began when I could not accept the admonition of the doctor there was no treatment available for this condition. I knew immediately in my heart that if there was nothing he as a doctor could do then it would be up to me. I could not accept this type of prognosis without putting up a fight. And so I did the only thing I knew to do.

For some time I had been following the AIDS story in the New York Native, the local gay newspaper, and had been keeping track of various experimental treatments being tried by those who were already ill. At this time there was much talk about a drug, Isoprinosine, believed to be helpful in rebuilding the immune system. Although it was widely available in Europe and Mexico, it was not available in the United States. It was also being used in conjunction with an antiviral drug Ribavirin, believed to prevent the reproduction of the virus.

Although the Ribavirin was responsible for some serious side effects, the Isoprinosine was not. The idea behind this treatment was that Ribavirin would halt the spread of the virus throughout the body while Isoprinosine would serve to rebuild immune function. Together, it was believed, these drugs could arrest and perhaps reverse the progress of AIDS.

I decided I must obtain Isoprinosine for both Wil and myself. We decided that the side effects of Ribavirin were too severe to take the risk at this early point in our illness. Rather than take the two drugs in combination we would take only the one.

A friend of mine from London had another friend who was working in an English pharmaceutical company. This firm was manufacturing the drug under the name of Immunovir. He had been supplying another friend of ours with this drug. Through our friend we were able to secure our own connection for the drugs. Within two weeks of receiving our dismal blood test results, a package arrived from London containing a three month supply of Isoprinosine for both Wil and myself. We began taking it immediately.

It is hard to describe the effect obtaining this medicine had for us. To be able to feel as if there were something one could take to help his condition was a tremendous relief. The helplessness engendered by being told there was nothing in the line of treatment available for this condition had all of the quality of a nightmare. It was as if one were being pursued by a killer virus from which there could be no escape. Each time you outfoxed it for a time it was again there over your shoulder, ready to devour you again. The desperate attempt to escape continued on endlessly without a chance of safety.

Later, I would come to understand totally the unsettling nightmarish quality of our dilemma. For now, the relief, whether justified or not, of having something tangible with which to treat ourselves provided us with some desperately needed ease from our distress.

SHUFFLE OFF TO MEXICO

We continued on with our life with as much normalcy as possible throughout the fall. With the exception of a few minor bouts with colds and minor fungal infections, there was not much that would outwardly reflect the tremendous inner tensions we were both under. Every news item that caught our eye pertaining to AIDS, however, only served to increase our growing inner paranoia. I would find myself neurotically checking every mole and spot on my body, searching for Kaposi lesions. As if the strain of dealing with this direct threat on our lives was not enough, the media was full of fear-filled accounts of the total fatality of this condition. In addition to this, there were increasing cries for all manner of sanctions against those with this disease and against the homosexual community at large.

If the medication we were taking provided us with any comfort, then even this was taken away by the realization that in addition to coping with our immediate health situation, we also had to cope with the knowledge that most of the world considered us a scourge on humanity at long last getting our just desserts. The deep seated hatred I felt directed at me from those who disapproved of my choice of who to love added to my growing despair. The realization dawned on me that the only thing making this time different from the dark ages was the degree of sophistication of our technology. The basic heart of man was as dark as ever. If my condition seemed to remain stable, my sense of security was becoming increasingly undermined.

As Christmas approached I became curious to see where I stood physically in terms of my blood profile. We had been taking isoprinosine for over three months and during this time our health appeared to be stable. I was secretly optimistic that the medicine had done its job and we had weathered the storm. We had exhausted our supply of pills and didn't want to invest even more money into buying the medicine if it was not needed. There were reports that the price of the pills was increasing rapidly.

We both had blood drawn and in addition, Wil called the doctor's attention to a bothersome spot appearing on his leg. The doctor took a biopsy. We went about our daily routines trying not to think of the impending results. On the 1st of December the results came in. Wil's blood profile remained unchanged from the previous test in September. My results, however, had taken a dramatic turn for the worst. My already depressed T-cell count had dropped in half. In addition, the biopsy on Wil's leg came back positive for Kaposi Sarcoma. Our anticipated reprieve had taken a cruel twist. The bottom had fallen out of our world.

As a haircolorist, the weeks leading up to the Christmas holiday are the busiest time of the year. In those few short weeks between Thanksgiving and New Years, it is as if every client you have ever serviced must be attended to. The sheer physical requirement to complete this task is at best difficult and, with the underlying strain of what I had been experiencing in my personal life, it was nearly incapacitating. I was torn between my professional responsibilities to my clientele and the need to pull back and feed that energy into myself.

Now, on top of all this, had come the diagnosis of Kaposi Sarcoma for Wil and the increasing disintegration of my own immune system. We felt our only hope at this point was to obtain the medicine Ribavirin from Mexico. The possibility of its toxic side effects no longer outweighed the immediate threat we were now facing. The Kaposi on Wil's leg would no longer allow us to pretend things were getting better.

We made reservations on Aero Mexico to fly to Mexico City

in two weeks. We felt the larger metropolitan area would offer us the maximum opportunity for finding the quantity of medicine we were seeking. Already we had heard reports of shortages and price gouging in the cities along the US-Mexican border, as more and more Americans turned southward, seeking relief. We felt our chances for success would be greatest in Mexico City.

Friday, December 13, 1985, was Wil's 40th birthday. That evening we attended a birthday party in Wil's honor at the home of his best friend Eric. The next morning we were scheduled to leave for Mexico City. The official story to the guests was that we were going to Acapulco for a few days rest. If anyone wondered why I would be leaving town in the midst of my busiest work season, they had too much tact to ask.

The night of the party was filled with such poignancy. We were both overwhelmed with the realization that this could possibly be the last birthday celebration we would have together. Yet the warmth felt that night, among the circle of our closest friends, helped to soothe the gnawing fears of our hearts. If fate decreed we were soon to die, at least we knew at this moment we were among people who loved and cared for us.

Early the next morning our adventure began. We knew what needed to be done and we were certain in our conviction that the success of this trip was our own responsibility. The dynamic tensions at work within us gave the whole affair a feeling of imminent danger and yet exciting adventure. Our adrenalin was certainly rushing.

We arrived in Mexico City early that Saturday afternoon, after a long and exhausting flight from New York City. After some problems in finding our luggage, we picked up our rented Volkswagen and headed for the hotel. The El Presidente Chapultapec was cool and modern, and there we found shelter from the dusty city and weariness of our journey.

That evening we left the hotel and began our search for the needed drugs. Not knowing much about the city, we began crisscrossing commercial areas looking for the signs announcing "la farmacia". To our delight, in no time we found a drugstore. What we quickly came to realize, however, was these drugstores stocked only one or two boxes each of the precious medication. One box was only one day's supply for one person. For the three month supply for each of us we hoped to find, we would need to visit dozens of pharmacies.

The next three days were spent in what seemed like an endless search for the needed drugs. I drove the car through the city's congested streets until we found a pharmacy. Then Wil would jump out and attempt to buy whatever Ribavirin was available. Slowly, box by box, we purchased the drugs we needed.

The seemingly endless ride through the narrow streets of Mexico City was dirty and tiring. The exhaust and the pollution burned my eyes. The tensions caused by the constant race against our limited stay, caused us to be on edge with each other. Wil became tired and was satisfied to leave with less medicine than we had planned to buy. I would not rest from the search, however. I pushed us to continue until finally I too could go no further.

The wee hours of the night before we were to return to New York were spent trying to consolidate our illegal booty into a more manageable size. There was no way we would be able to pass through customs with so many boxes of pills. Each box contained one dozen pills wrapped in vacuum packed foil. It was little more than one day's supply in each box and we had enough boxes for a three month supply for each of us. We emptied the contents of each box. We then wrapped the foil strips in stacks of ten each and bound them tightly with masking tape to compress them into a smaller size.

Each stack was then carefully hidden throughout our luggage. Some were packed in shoes, some folded into pants and shirts, some stuffed into jacket pockets, and some wrapped with dirty underwear and socks. If we were searched carefully by customs, there was scarcely a prayer we would pass through undetected. If their inspection was casual, we would be fine. We really had no choice and so were resolved to do what we had to do.

We made contingency plans in case one of us was discovered and the other passed through undetected. I wanted Wil to go through first. If he made it into the country safely, I would then follow. If I were caught, I wanted him to leave me there and first take the medicine home. Then he could return and bail me out. He refused. He felt if one of us was caught, we would be arrested together. He would not leave me in custody alone.

On arrival at JFK in New York, Wil and I were separated from each other. He was carrying only a birth certificate and was required to go through a separate procedure from those of us with passports. I had to proceed to the luggage claim area alone. There I waited for our luggage to appear and for Wil to clear inspection. My wait seemed like an eternity. Finally, I saw him through the crowd and relief rushed through my body. We proceeded through customs together. The officer asked but a few brief questions about the reason for our visit to Mexico, and then waved us through the gate. We passed over into freedom.

In my pocket was the phone number of a friend who worked in the media for NBC. If I had been arrested, my first call would have been to her. I wanted the world to know our government would take medicine from the hands of the dying. Our anger and frustration at the experiences of the last few days bubbled to the surface. We went home and had a long hard cry.

We were also angry at ourselves, angry for having caught this disease in the first place and for having put ourselves in this position. We felt dirty, ashamed, and afraid.

A CHRISTMAS GIFT

Christmas 1985 was upon us now. I was starting to feel as if this would be my last chance ever to celebrate this holiday. With the way things were going I wasn't so sure either one of us would be around at this same time next year.

It had been several years since I had been home for the Christmas holidays. I had always allowed my work to keep me in New York. Since Wil's parents lived in nearby New Rochelle, we had always spent the holiday there with them.

But this year was different. Faced with a future that seemed ever more menacing, I wanted to have one more chance to spend Christmas with my own family. Wil had never been to my home town or my parents' house and it was important for me to be able to share these places from my past with him. He agreed to come along with me.

Wil had never met my father. Although he had spent time with my mother on several occasions, he had only heard stories from me about my father. My father and I had a rather uneasy relationship in my childhood years and although to some degree we had smoothed out the rough edges of our relationship, it was still one in which I was not totally comfortable. I held considerable resentment toward him for what I considered to be his abusive treatment of my mother and myself.

Due to my strict upbringing in the Church of the Nazarene, a small fundamentalist denomination, I had never been fully comfortable with my father. As an alcoholic, he represented to me everything the church taught it was wrong for a person to be. As an impressionable child, I had accepted these judgments and projected them onto him without fully realizing what I was doing. Only later would I come to understand the role these judgments were playing in my own illness.

All through my youthful years at home, I had increasingly shut down any communication with my father and was unable to sustain a loving relationship with him. I felt he did not fully approve of my artistic inclinations and that he was embarrassed by my lack of interest in sports and other outdoor activities. Because these things had never been expressed, they still stood like an invisible wall between us. Passing time had slowly broken the wall down, but it still remained there to a large degree.

I wanted Wil to meet my father. I felt until they met, there would be a part of me Wil could not understand fully. In the present circumstance, this was most important to me.

Christmas day arrived and we flew to Florida to be with my family. Everyone gathered at my mother's house to exchange presents and share Christmas dinner. I had bought an electric train for my six year old nephew and because it was complicated to assemble, Wil and I helped him to set it up. After a short time, however, I lost interest in the project. It was tedious and time consuming. Alone, Wil continued to set up the tiny track and the accessories we had purchased to go with it. For several hours, he patiently worked with the train set until it was completely assembled. He then took time to show my nephew how to use it. Unbeknownst to me, my father had been observing Wil the entire time. He noticed how we all lost interest in assembling the train set. He had seen how Wil patiently continued working until it was entirely assembled. Wil's willingness to continue through with this tedious task until it was finished, for a child not even his own relative, did not go unnoticed by my father. This one act was enough for my father to accept Wil totally.

From this point on, Wil and my father became very close. My father shared all his stories from "the good old days" with Wil.

Wil, on the other hand, was completely charmed by my father's country simplicity and his stories about a part of American life to which he had never been exposed. They seemed to enjoy each other's company immensely. If I hadn't been so delighted in seeing these two important men in my life enjoying each other's company so much, I would have probably been jealous.

Instead, I was able to learn a lot about my father that Christmas holiday. I had never seen him as animated as he was that day. Wil had drawn him out of himself in a way I had seldom seen before. As I observed him I was impressed by his sensitivity to what was real about life. As I continued to listen, I was able to recognize many of the judgments I had held against him for so long. For the first time in a long while I was feeling affection for my father. This was a shift that did not fail to catch my attention. In facing my own mortality, I too was beginning to appreciate the difference between what was important and real and what was not. Maybe it was possible we had things in common after all.

Wil and I left for New York the next day after having spent a wonderful time together with my family. As far as my relationship with my father was concerned, the old wound in my heart felt much, much better. This was a gift I had not expected. I had seen a side of him I had never seen before. It was the same side of myself I was becoming increasingly aware of through my own struggle for life - a struggle beginning to take on a paradoxical mixture of pain and pleasure. At the strangest, time in the midst of all the trauma, there would appear an unexpected gift.

Although the prospect of facing death now seemed to hover over my entire life like a menacing cloud, at the most improbable times an occasional ray of light would break through the impenetrable darkness and illuminate the rich texture of my life. Something was revealed that I had overlooked in the past. Increasingly I was beginning to feel a faint stirring within myself on levels I had not had the courage to explore before. AIDS was beginning to reveal a dimension of life previously obscure to me. Yet it was uncomfortable to think this experience could possibly have anything of value to offer. What good thing could possibly come from AIDS?

The winter that followed was a time of intensifying panic. My fears about what was happening to my body seemed to be justified by the slow deterioration of my physical condition. Although I had exhibited no major AIDS-related infections, I had increasingly been plagued by numerous fungal infections. My tongue had grown a coat for the winter. I was suffering from leukoplakia. My propensity for colds and flus, as well as a general sense of dis-ease, seemed to increase.

Internalization of my fear led to the formation of a stomach ulcer, causing extremely uncomfortable symptoms. I would go to work feeling perfectly well, and before I could finish my first client, I would become violently ill and begin to vomit uncontrollably. The first time this happened I thought I had food poisoning. But as it continued to happen day after day, it became obvious there was another problem. My doctor put me on tranquilizers to calm my nerves and to help alleviate the symptoms.

Later this ulcer would come back to serve me in a powerful way. It would give me a personal example of the impact of a fearful mind upon the body. But for now it served only to terrorize me further.

Late in January I developed a flu which threatened to become pneumonia and was laid up in bed for a period of well over two weeks. This allowed me a great deal of time with myself. It was during this stay in bed that I decided to write my life story. I was sure I was facing death and if my life was not long on quantity, I knew at the very least I had some unusual stories to tell.

I began to write. I started with my birth and diligently continued day after day to put my memories down on paper. When Wil would come home after work, I would read him my day's effort. He always enjoyed the stories and felt I had a natural talent for expressing myself through writing. He urged me to stay with it. Encouraged, I continued to write.

For the next two weeks I continued to pour out my life's story on paper until I had written about my life up to the age of

26. By this time I was finally beginning to recover from my flu. The time was approaching for me to return to work. I gradually lost interest in continuing with my writing, convincing myself no one would want to read it anyway. As I settled back into my work routine I stopped completely.

I was unaware of it at the time but the writing down of my early life experience began a dramatic psychological shift in the way I perceived myself and my life. The deeper currents of my familial relationships became obvious on paper, in ways my memory failed to reveal. I saw with clarity my own role in the alienation I felt from my father.

I could see more of the dynamics of our relationship. If blame were to be placed for our breakdown in communication, it would have to be shared equally between us. For the first time I was left to consider how it must have felt to have a child that withheld his love. On a certain level I could see this is what I had done. My heart began to soften around the memory of my childhood.

By acting on the intuitive hunch to write down my life story, I had set in motion a process much larger than I could imagine at the time. Writing had unleashed memories and images of my past deeply buried in my unconscious. One by one they now came into remembrance. These memories were laying the groundwork for my own healing. On a conscious level, however, I was not yet aware of what was happening.

MY AWAKENING

As March approached, our supply of the precious medicines was beginning to dwindle. Not wanting there to be an interruption in our intake of pills, we planned to return to Mexico once again. To relieve some of the stress of the trip we planned a 5 day trip to the beach at Cancun before we were to continue on to Mexico City. We wanted to get away from the reality of our life struggle in New York and just allow ourselves time off from what was happening there.

Before we were to leave, our good friend Bill Sullivan recommended we pick up a book and take it along with us on our trip. Bill had been diagnosed with cancer over ten years previously and had been free of the disease for some time. The name of the book was "GETTING WELL AGAIN" by Simonton and Simonton. It was a book about the work of two doctors involving the connection of mind and body in the process of healing cancer. Through the use of visualization and other techniques varying degrees of remission had been achieved by their patients.

I accompanied Wil to the bookstore to purchase this book and while waiting for him I glanced through some nearby shelves. A book from the Metaphysical and Occult section caught my eye and drew me toward it. It was a book on the work of Edgar Cayce involving religion and psychic phenomena.

I had heard of Edgar Cayce's work and had been interested in paranormal phenomena for some time. The title linking psychic phenomena to religious experience was more than I could resist.

Many years earlier I had experienced an out-of-body experience and had believed ever since in the existence of consciousness exclusive of the physical body. As a youth, however, my upbringing had been in a narrow fundamentalist context of God which I had long since rejected. The subject matter of the book was too intriguing for me to pass up. What could one topic possibly have to do with the other? I purchased the book and took it to Mexico to read as I relaxed at the beach.

The five days beside the clear warm waters of the Caribbean Sea did a lot to soothe what were now almost permanently jangled nerves and served to lift me up and away from the events of my life as they continued to unfold in New York. It was there, sitting in the warm tropical sun, that I began reading the books which would in time alter the course of my illness and my entire life.

I began with the book on Edgar Cayce and continued until I had completed the Simonton book. It was through reading these two books that I became aware for the first time of the role of the mind and attitude on the health of the body, and the relationship between psychic phenomena and deep spiritual experience.

For the first twenty years of my life I had been raised under the strict teaching of the Bible as interpreted through the doctrine of the Church of the Nazarene, a small fundamentalist sect of Christianity. The God I learned of there was a jealous, vengeful, sovereign who demanded unquestioning adoration and obedience. It was a God who stood ever ready to punish the slightest infraction of what seemed in my mind to be an impossible standard. When I was a child God seemed like an unpleasable tyrant and I grew up with a sense of guilt about myself which I could never quite put my finger on.

With the onset of puberty and the dawning realization that I was less than totally heterosexual, what had been only a vague sense of guilt now became quite clear. Not only was my awakening sexuality an energy to be suppressed and denied until some future date when I was safely married, but it was then to be allowed only in the context of conceiving a child. It was never to be indulged in for the sheer pleasure it seemed to promise.

As for the growing awareness of my sexual attraction to members of my own sex, this was truly a cross to bear. Here I was, created with the desire for another of my own sex and then forbidden to indulge in those desires lest I burn in hell forever. To express an aspect of my God-given nature was, in some way that was unclear to me, an abomination to the God who had given it to me. It was the ultimate "catch-22."

Time after time I made serious attempts to turn my life and will over to His service out of fear of the flames of hell. Fear was the only motivation I ever learned. Finally, finding the task more than I could ever hope to accomplish, and God's supposed love and support nowhere to be found, I decided if I was dammed already I might as well forget Him and enjoy the time I had remaining on this earth. And so I rejected this angry God and Christainity as I had been taught it, and let those issues fall away from my life. As the years ensued, whenever a question of a religious nature concerning these issues would enter my mind I would push it away, knowing that the God I had learned of just couldn't be real. If He were, I would have rather have gone to hell than subjugate myself to such a tyrant. Heaven with Him would definitely have been hell for me. For those reasons I lived the next 13 years of my life with no conscious awareness of God, the sole source of strength in my life being my own self.

There was a problem with this approach which I was unaware of at the time, however. I was throwing out the baby of my spirituality with the bath water of religion. Instead of pushing these ideas away from me what I really needed to do was examine them more closely. I needed to clearly see these distorted ideas about God and myself for what they were. They needed to be replaced with clearer truths that would support and validate me as a human being. Instead, I was afraid of what I might find inside, and could not bear to look within. I unknowingly shoved these twisted ideas deep within my subconscious. I threw away my real and necessary spirituality in the rush to rid myself of this damning religious teaching.

Several years later I moved to New York in search of the sense of acceptance that always seemed to elude me. It was there that I created a successful career for myself, acquiring the income I felt I needed in order to build an image of myself worthy of love. I used all the things money could buy to build barriers between myself and others. I wanted to prevent them from seeing what I feared to be the truth about myself. I closed off my heart, refusing to let anyone in, believing I could protect myself from the over-whelming pain of rejection. Little did I realize I was the one being shut off from love.

It was for these reasons that Edgar Cayce was to play such a large role in changing the course of my life. He was to show me that in turning within, in search of my own deepest knowledge, I was unknowingly turning toward God.

Edgar Cayce was a trance channel known as "the sleeping prophet". While in an unconscious trance state, he channeled a tremendous volume of information on a broad range of topics, from physical healing treatments to an outlook on Christainity and the Bible large enough to include reincarnation and karma. His inter-pretations of the symbology of the Bible reached far beyond the written words and pulled forward the deeper truths upon which the words rested.

During Cayce's lifetime many people sought his help in their quest for healings of all kinds. More often than not he would deal with their illness and wellness not just in terms of what needed to be done on a physical level, but in terms of the change of mind and attitude without which there could be no healing of the body. In many cases he would not address the physical ailment directly at all, rather he would deal specifically with the mental aspects of the illness. At other times he would speak of present-day illness in terms of influences from the patient's previous lifetimes on earth. Over and over he refused to separate the body from the mind as in current medical thought.

Rather than these ideas being totally new to me, it was as

if I were being reminded of something long since forgotten. I had never before heard these ideas articulated in just such a way as this, however. Here were people being given mental solutions to physical problems that had defied all conventional efforts toward healing, and yet they were being healed. They were, however, being guided into greater avenues of self-awareness in order for the healing to occur.

As I lay there on the beach in Mexico, I let these ideas play through my mind in relaxed contemplation, much like the sunlight dancing on the clear waters of the Caribbean before me. Ever so slightly I began to open up my mind to the idea that perhaps in my own experience with AIDS it was going to be necessary for me to expand my search beyond the seeking for just a physical solution. Indeed, the medical profession itself was the first to admit they had no answers for the disease, and I was the first to question the effectiveness of the medicines I was so desperately seeking.

Perhaps if Edgar Cayce had been there to do a reading for me he would have pointed out my own need to deal with the mental and spiritual aspects of my illness. Although this was not possible, since he was long since dead, in my heart I knew this would have been the case. I was going to have to open up new doors if I was to find the answer I was looking for.

The remainder of the trip to Mexico City accomplished what it was intended for. Wil and I were able to obtain more of the precious medicines we needed. I returned to New York with a new thirst, however. This thirst was to read every book on Edgar Cayce and his work I could get my hands on. I was not to be disappointed either. My search of a nearby metaphysical bookstore turned up at least ten such books. I bought them all, took them home, and began to read.

Much of the work of Edgar Cayce centered around the teachings of Christianity and the Bible. While in trance he would expound on various ideas found within the Bible, but the outlook on Christianity he espoused was much broader than the narrow fundamentalist view I had been exposed to as a child. He incor-

porated concepts of karma and reincarnation into the more traditional Christian teachings, expanding them into a greater
understanding.

Of God, Cayce, said, "There is no punishing God." There
was only a God of mercy and allowance. On first encountering this
idea I could not even comprehend it. With the distorted view of
God I had held, this was an impossibility. If God was not going
to punish you when you were bad, what was the point? It seemed
like so much wishful thinking to me.

As I continued to study the material, however, I began to
discover a God in which there was no judgment. Even forgiveness
was unnecessary with this God, for in his eyes there had never been
a judgment of guilt. There was only an incredible ongoing love and
allowance for life. The Cayce material said any judgment that
seemed to be occurring was not a punishment from an avenging
God but was something happening in my own mind. Therefore,
it was only there, in my own mind, that forgiveness needed to occur.
Salvation was as simple as forgiving oneself!

This was definitely not the wrathful God of my childhood.
These ideas spoke to me of something so much greater, so much
less fearful. I was not a person unwilling to look at my own
judgments and failures. Nor was I unwilling to extend mercy and
forgiveness to myself. Could an eternal God without beginning
or end be so petty as to damn me eternally for something I did
in the span of a few short years? I knew in that one simple moment
of realization that the treacherous God of my childhood was not
the truth at all. Instead the idea of God had been resurrected as
a living, loving presence in the temple of my own heart. I was filled
with an incredible sense of relief.

The material went on to explain it was the law of karma,
of cause and effect, that was responsible for creating the events in
one's life. Cayce described it as a constant "meeting of the self".
He taught that in the body of our life, relationships, and events
we experience, we have reflected back to us the ideas and attitudes
about life and ourselves which we hold within our own conscious-

ness. If something in our experience seems to be a punishment, in truth it is merely a reflection of our own distorted ideas about life. Its purpose is simply to bring us to a clearer understanding. Recognizing this, we can choose to lovingly face the event for what it has to teach us about ourselves. We can change our minds and in doing so release the experience. This, Cayce said, was the exercise of free will - the choice to think as we choose about the events of our lives. In facing life with love for the lesson it seeks to teach, karma is transmuted by loving acceptance. The need for the experience will be no more. It can then leave our life.

Through these teachings I began to awaken to the idea that I was neither the innocent victim of a deadly virus nor the recipient of a damning punishment from an angry God. Rather I had before me, in the form of AIDS, a self-created lesson I could either accept as "a millstone around my neck or a stepping stone to greater glory." I knew my illness was indeed a tremendous millstone and yet I was beginning to see that if I was willing to face it and accept the lessons and changes it sought to bring me, I could indeed transform it into a stepping stone of equal glory. I had always been quick to claim responsibility for the successes in my life. I was now being asked to take responsibility for the things I judged failures.

Quickly the realization was dawning on me that there was nothing I was presented with in life to which I was not given a way out. I realized for the first time that if I were willing to face the lesson before me, I could defy the medical profession and release this experience. The Cayce readings had filled my heart with the greatest hunger I had ever known, to establish my connection with my own true identity. They had given me a glimmer of a reality greater than I had ever imagined.

Through continuing study of many different metaphysical works I came to realize that "the mind that was in Christ" is the same mind in each one of us. It is a level of understanding deep within where the limitation of human experience intersects with the unlimited potential of our divinity. It is a level undistorted by the judgments of the ego personality.

I began to see beyond the veil modern Christainity had thrown around the messenger, Jesus, to the truth of the message he brought. It is each one of us who is a son of God, the human expression of a limitless reality, and Jesus is our elder brother. He came to show the way to a sleeping humanity, ignorant of its true identity. Instead they worshiped the messenger and forgot the message. "The kingdom of heaven is within". My heart began to resonate to the impossibly wonderful truth of it all!

My knowledge of the Bible was still quite solid. One by one all the verses I had learned in Sunday school over all those early years came rushing back to me. I now understood them in a new way and was overwhelmed that their meaning would suddenly have so much reality for me. Now they were not just words but had real meaning to me in ways that had validity in my own life. A sense of excitement and joy began to swell within my heart and I knew without a doubt at the deepest levels of my being that I was on to the truth about myself and my life - the Truth that would indeed set me free!

I was realizing for the first time that at the most basic level I had sold my own self short. I didn't even know who I was! I was not just a biological creature as science had said and my life was not an accident with no meaning or purpose. I was literally a son of God, the Christ, with an energy system within my physical body for attunement to ALL THAT IS. I cried in realization of my true identity. I knew it was true! My heart swelled with joy at the thought.

I had to make a decision. If these ideas were so, then they would have to be something I could make real for myself. They would have to be more than an abstract belief in a hoped for plan of salvation. There would have to be a realization I could feel in the deepest recesses of my heart and demonstrate at least to a degree in my life. In that moment I made a choice. I would seek to know the truth about myself and my connection to the universal source.

Edgar Cayce talked in detail of the symbology of the stories in the Bible. One that impressed me as relevant to myself concerned the story of Jesus as he prayed in the garden of Gesthsemane before he was to be crucified. Edgar Cayce spoke of the symbology of the prayer "not my will, but thine", the importance of surrendering self will to the will of God. He explained that healing was not something we could force to happen, rather it is the natural course of things we need to step back from and allow to occur.

If one cuts his finger it is not necessary to visualize the action of the red and white blood cells in order for the cut to heal. There is an intelligence in the body with a propensity toward healing. Unless we pick at the cut, with time it will heal unassisted. With all illness it is necessary only to remove the mental and physical irritations blocking the natural state of health for healing to occur. This healing is not something we make happen. Instead we step aside and allow the process to follow its natural course.

It was totally clear at this point in my search for healing that my ego mind had no answers left for me. I knew my life and health had long before spun out of my conscious control. There were no doctors to turn to for a magic pill. The struggle was no longer worth the pain. There was no where left to turn but within.

I still wasn't totally sure what God was and I didn't really know how to pray. I didn't have any clear idea how I could begin to claim my promised birthright of health and peace. I did know I could pray for guidance not to an old man on a cloud but to a living reality existing within my own being. In recognition of my own inadequacy and with the most sincere plea of my life, I knelt in the middle of my living room floor and uttered this prayer..."Dear God, I don't want to die, but I don't really care anymore. I have struggled against death as long as I care to struggle. I know there is a reason for what is happening to me and if I could just learn what it is all about, I am willing to know. I just don't want to die not knowing what this is all about. Nevertheless, not my will, but thine!"

I began to cry, quietly at first, then growing in intensity until I could feel it coursing in waves throughout my entire body. The tears ran down my face, wetting the floor on which I lay and then finally ran dry. Through those tears I relinquished all control of my illness. I didn't know what was to come from all this, but I knew it was out of my hands now. I sighed in relief.

The lessons yet to come in my life appeared very rapidly from this point in time. It was as if the teacher, or the book, or the experience necessary for my growth and development seemed to surface from out of nowhere. I continued with my study of the Cayce material and for the first time began to follow a daily practice of prayer and meditation. To allow myself the time for all this I began to awaken an hour earlier each morning so I would have time for meditation before I began my regular day.

At first it seemed as if I were just sitting in my dark living room alone, waiting for something to happen that never did, but gradually over time and with persistent practice I learned to still my untrained mind, to let go of everything around me, and to allow myself to reach deeply into the stillness of my own inner being. There I began for the first time to get in touch with the deepest levels of my feelings. I began to spend time in contemplation on the concept of oneness and other ideas I was reading about and wanted to understand more fully. Slowly I began to fathom the implications of just what the interrelatedness of all life truly means. I began to see more clearly what my relationship was to the whole of life. I began to know I was not alone.

As time passed little light bulbs began to go off in my head at the strangest times and I would know something I hadn't known before. It was as if new ideas and understandings would enter my mind from out of the blue. I knew this was somehow connected to my morning meditations and it gave me the encouragement I needed to press ahead with my inner connection and the faith to know that there the answers lay.

As the awareness of my true self slowly began to penetrate my personal darkness, my growing sense of self-love became reflected in my treatment and attitude toward my body. It was important that my desire to live be translated into concrete physical actions. If I really desired to live then I had to question why I continued to put foods and drugs into my body that interfered with its optimum functioning. I now began a program to detoxify and nourish my ailing body. I implemented a cleansing diet of fruit and juices and began to study the concept of food combining. On a daily basis I spent time carefully selecting the fresh fruits and vegetables that would be my food for that day. No longer did I continue to eat out in restaurants every night but began preparing my own meals at home. I began to nourish myself and to show love and respect for my body through these physical acts. I began to search into many new areas exploring new approaches to healing.

For the first time I sought out the assistance of a chiropractor to help me release the considerable tension I held in my back and shoulders. I wanted my spine realigned so the energies of life could flow unimpeded through my body. I began a series of weekly massages. If the body was an instrument for attunement to the universal mind as Cayce said, then I was determined I would do all in my power to make mine totally functional.

At this point it was not so much that I wanted to attack my illness, but rather I was seeking to know just who I really am. "Seek Ye first the kingdom of God and his righteousness and all these things shall be added unto You" had a new meaning for me. I knew my health would not come as a result of fighting my illness, but rather as a by-product of seeking my connection to the power within me. I knew my illness was not about the physical body so much as it was about the pain in my soul. My health was simply reflecting my attitudes about myself and life. I now knew the kingdom of heaven was within and was a deep level of peace and joy that comes from understanding who you really are. I surrendered the physical result and sought instead to heal my broken heart.

My growing commitment to the search for the truth of my identity became the consuming focus of my life. If any of my friends had failed to notice a change in me up until this time, it was impossible for them to ignore it now. In my new found enthusiasm for loving, I was quick to share my experiences and ideas with them whether they were interested or not. I'm sure more than one of my friends pulled away from me, not understanding how such things could be coming from my mouth. They had known my life before and I myself would have flinched in embarrassment on hearing the words that now so freely came from my lips. Undaunted, I committed myself to my quest more deeply than ever.

I wanted so much to share with Wil my excitement over these new understandings, but the more he would hear the word God, the more he would resist the things I would tell him. Spirituality was something he had long since rejected along with his Catholic upbringing and it was something his scientific mind was not about to reconsider. My insistence only served to intensify his resistance to these ideas. Finally I came to realize the impossibility of making another person understand a truth by telling it to them. Only through a personal demonstration in one's own life can others come to see what is real. I resolved even more deeply to pursue the path that stretched out before me. I vowed to myself I would rise above the self-accepted limitations of human consciousness about AIDS and in doing so light the way for Wil.

A SCIENTIFIC APPROACH

While the teachings of Edgar Cayce had sent me in a metaphysical direction in my quest for healing, it was a direction in which Wil had not the slightest interest. In fact any mention of God or Christ or any reference to psychic phenomena sent him running in the opposite direction. In his mind these things were just so much superstition. If there was to be any road toward healing for him it would have to be a scientific one.

Wil had a degree in electrical engineering and his vocation at the time was that of a computer programmer. Not only was he of Catholic Hispanic background but he had been a Captain in the U.S. Air Force. His mind-set was a rigid one that dealt with concrete facts, not faith. Before he would venture a trip across the room he would first plot his course, back it up with a few alternate routes, and then begin the journey. He left nothing to chance or spontaneity. Any belief in God had been left behind long ago.

It was for these reasons that the Simonton book dealing with experimental cancer treatments was to make such an impression on him. The book was written in two parts. The first part of the book dealt with case histories of people who had been diagnosed with terminal cancer and had been given up for dead by their doctors. Yet in case after case tumors shrank and disappeared and dying patients had completely recovered against all odds.

The second part of the book dealt with the controversial techniques that had been employed by these patients in their recovery. They had used techniques such as dream interpretation, deep healing imagery, visualization, and meditation. These therapies were used in conjunction with conventional medical treatment.

For Wil, the second part of the book was too far out for his scientific mind to accept. These new therapies had no scientific validity in his eyes. The first part of the book was different, however. Here in case study after case study were people faced with a fatal prognosis yet able to reverse the outcome. In the case of two people facing a similar diagnosis, one would succumb to the disease and yet the other was able to beat seemingly unbeatable odds and recover health. It was this part of the book he was unable to ignore. These case histories it presented were documented facts. To Wil's mind this was the kind of evidence he needed before he would begin his own exploration of just what was behind these recoveries.

After reading the book it suddenly occurred to him that if he were able to construct a computer model of just what were the characteristics of a surviving cancer patient he could then apply what he had found to AIDS. He knew there was a lot being written about people recovering from cancer, but there was nothing of this type of information about people with AIDS. On a very gut level he knew there was no such thing as a germ or virus that kills everyone who becomes infected by it. Perhaps he could use what he would learn in his search for a solution to his own predicament. It made sense. After all, in 1985 the medical profession was quick to point out there was nothing they could do for AIDS. There was nothing to loose.

Wil returned to New York with a desire to read more books of this nature. In contrast to my own desire to read metaphysical books on spiritual healing, Wil was drawn to books of dry factual case studies written by psychiatrists and behavioral scientists. Nights in New York found us side-by-side in bed, each with a stack of books of our own choosing on our respective night tables.

As turned off as Wil was to my approach, so too did I find his books boring and dry. The important thing was, however, that in spite of the differences in our directions, we each allowed the other his own approach to the problem before us. One of the strengths of our relationship had always been that we had never tried to force on one another our own pictures of how things should be done. We loved each other for the way we really were, not trying to change each other to fit our mold.

For this reason our paths to healing seemed to diverge in completely opposite directions - Wil looking toward science for the answers and me looking within. Little did we dream at that point in time how our paths would come full-circle and meet at the point of healing. Such a thing seemed like an impossibly distant point in the future from our present perspective. It was one that was closer, however, than we could then know.

As Wil delved into the various books on case histories of cancer patients he began to see certain common threads shared by most of the survivors. Certain attributes and attitudes seemed to set them apart from the more typical patients who were succumbing to the disease. It was from these attributes he began to build an emerging profile of a survivor.

First and foremost on the list he found a refusal by the patient to accept the fatality of the illness. It was not that they refused to accept the disease, rather they did not believe that the outcome necessarily resulted in death. It was this attitude that allowed the patient to react in a positive manner, seeking for a solution to the illness. On the other hand, those accepting the fatality of their condition usually resigned themselves to death and did not seek any other treatment. When hope was taken away, there was no will to resist the prognosis. Without hope, no search for a solution was undertaken.

Secondly, all the people who were surviving had a real commitment to life. They seemed to feel they had a purpose and a reason for living. All of the patients when asked, claimed they wanted to get well. Many of them, however, had nothing to get well for. Health for them meant going back to a job they hated or a relationship in which they were not happy. The people who were recovering had things in their lives yet to accomplish which

/ 39

ɔrtant. One woman who later recovered, when told ɔnths to live, laughed. She said she had five small children... ɨad no intention of dying until they were grown and through with college.

Thirdly, it seemed to Wil that the meaner the patient, the more likely their recovery. This was puzzling at first. It appeared maybe the old expression "Only the good die young" wasn't so far from the truth. On further examination however, he began to see it was not meanness that was the key to survival. Rather, it was the willingness of the patient to express his anger and discomfort and to complain when he felt like it, that made him appear to others to be mean. The meek patient on the other hand, who never complained and was regarded by the doctors and nurses as an ideal patient, was not recovering.

This meek patient was not allowing himself to fully feel or express his feelings about the illness. In the face of a death sentence he was unable to express anger at having his life cut short. This patient had placed many restrictions on what he found acceptable to feel. Since these feelings were not being voiced outwardly they were instead being turned inwardly and expressed within the body. These repressed feelings were contributing to immune dysfunction and the disease process.

Lastly, the patient who had a certain reputation for stubbornness and was cited by the doctors and nurses as a difficult patient, tended to be among those that survived. These were patients who refused to blindly accept treatment or medication. Instead they wanted to know both the benefits and the drawbacks involved in any therapies they were to be given. They insisted on participating with their doctors in their own treatment. They refused to turn themselves over totally to the doctor to be fixed. Instead they questioned and researched the doctor's proposals and in the end would accept no treatment that went against their own inner guidance. They had a great deal of trust in themselves.

As Wil continued deeper into medical literature in his quest for more answers, it was not long before he came upon a new science.

It was a science that had been around for some 40 years or more and was in recent time gaining more and more credibility among current medical thought. It was, however, a science that was new to him. Its name was Psychoneuroimmunology - PNI. It was, to be more precise, the study of the impact of the mind on the function of the immune system. Here was scientifically documented evidence of the mind-body connection. This was no fluff psychology piece about positive thinking in some woman's magazine. This was concrete scientific data that said your thoughts and feelings had physical ramifications in the physical body. Through complex neurological and glandular reaction, emotion and attitude were translated into physical reality.

This was information Wil's rational approach could utilize. Here was an entire body of scientific data verifying the connection between the mind and the body. Finally he had discovered evidence to convince himself that what you think has consequences. This evidence provided him with the connecting link showing how the surviving attitudes he had compiled earlier were able to impact the physical body. It was an idea he had heard from me many times before, but was unable to accept because of my approach based on intuitive understanding. However, now that he had found scientific verification he could justify utilizing these ideas for himself.

In looking for evidence of the mind-body connection in his own life, Wil began to see examples everywhere. For instance, someone gives you a compliment and you blush in reaction. What just happened there? Blood moved through your body and collected in your face. A clear physical reaction. However, it was not the words causing this reaction. No, the words of themselves have no power. It was the individual interpretation of what was said that caused the body to react. The words of themselves were meaningless.

In a theater, a chilling murder is committed on the screen. Your skin responds by raising into goose bumps. Did the projection cause this reaction? Again no. The image itself is powerless. It is the reaction of your thoughts and feelings to the image.

Everywhere, examples from everyday life became clear to

him and began to confirm how thought impacts the physical body. It was no longer possible for him to discount the validity of this precept in relation to his own experience. He began to look more closely at the particulars of his own life in light of this new understanding.

It became clear that in order for this information to be of any use he was going to have to deal with his feelings. It was going to be necessary to take responsibility for the way he was feeling and find a way to change his reaction to situations that caused him stress. Denial as a coping-mechanism was no longer a viable option. By now he knew feelings have to be expressed. When they are not expressed outwardly, the evidence was suggesting, they were being expressed inwardly through complex biological processes. He was going to have to find a way to change anger and frustration into peace and joy. It seemed like a monumental task.

Wil was always a person that bartered for love. On a deep level he had accepted that in order for him to receive love, there was something he had to do to earn it. It had never occurred to him that he deserved love just because he existed. Love to him was a conditional thing.

He had always considered himself a good person, and because he was a good person he always did good deeds. It was not always because he really wanted to however. He did them because that's how he bartered for love.

At this time I was beginning to explore a wide variety of information. I was beginning to understand the role the mind plays in the creation of experience, and embrace the idea that beliefs create reality. For me this was a time of intense excitement as I was slowly coming to realize the role I had played in my own illness. I was understanding clearly these ideas were not about guilt but were about awakening to the tools that were inherent within me. I could make different choices and make changes in situations I had previously believed I had no effect upon. I was coming to realize I had resources at my disposal beyond my wildest dreams.

I felt I had to share these ideas with Wil. They offered a

piece of the puzzle he was missing. The problem was most of the information was from channeled sources. In Wil's mind this was not an acceptable source of information. As a last resort I used his need to please me in his own behalf. I pleaded with him to read some of the information. Because he felt he needed to do something for me to keep my approval, he reluctantly agreed to read just one book of my choosing.

The book I asked him to read was a very long one. It was a book that had been channeled through a trance medium and dealt with the role of belief in creation of personal reality. It was called "The Nature of Personal Reality" by Jane Roberts. The book was long and repetitious and for Wil it took several months of my steady coaxing to move him through it. It was a book, however, that was to change forever how he viewed information and it was to provide him with the missing link of how he could change his own beliefs.

The book was written in successive sections of material, dictated through the medium by the disembodied author named Seth. In addition there were personal comments and insights added by the medium herself. For Wil the medium reflected just about every judgment he held about people involved in psychic phenomena. He found her and her "insight" more the rambling of a schizoid mind. He considered her the ultimate "air head". But the part of the book that was channeled had a tremendous appeal. Here were powerful understandings of the workings of the mind delivered in a highly rational and convincing manner. It was information he responded to on a very gut level and yet it was coming from what he found to be a totally objectionable source. Here was a woman from a small town in upstate New York delivering information in trance that science was just beginning to discover.

Wil's experience with this book changed forever the way he would view information in the future. Never again would he be able to discount information because of its source. He realized for the first time that the source no longer had any real significance. It was how he reacted intuitively to the information that was the only thing of any real importance. This was a tremendous shift in his understanding. It flung open wide the doors to an expanded awareness of life. Through these doors he cautiously stepped.

The channeled information provided Wil with what had been up until this time the missing link in the workings of the mind-body connection. It gave him a basic understanding of how the emotional body is created by belief systems held in the individual consciousness.

Wil was discovering how his emotional reaction to an external event could be used as a marker to locate beliefs held in his own consciousness, beliefs that were the emotion's source. Beliefs could be located simply by the awareness of the feelings they were producing. Upon discovering the belief creating the reaction, a decision could be made to change the belief depending on the impact its resulting feeling was producing within the physical body.

Using this technique Wil began to explore his own belief systems. He was looking for unconscious ideas that were causing him to continually react in a negative way to many different situations he was encountering in his life. He began to see he was living his life under a tremendous number of "shoulds". These "shoulds" were causing him to experience anxiety, frustration, and anger. He discovered these "shoulds" caused him to try and control each situation which failed to meet his expectations of how it should be. He was constantly being forced to fix things. This was causing a tremendous amount of stress.

At this point Wil had learned enough about the physical impact of stress on the immune system to know he wanted to change his mind concerning some of the ideas he held about how things should be. He sought to simply allow things to be as they were. He also knew it had been scientifically documented that feelings of love, joy, and laughter could produce substances in the body that were not only natural pain killers, but were known to enhance immune functioning. In order to rebuild his own immune system he was going to have to change his mind to a point where he could begin to experience life in another way. Every belief causing him to experience less than joy was going to have to go.

When a child is young it has an unlimited view of life. There is nothing in the child's mind that is not in the realm of possibility for it. Life is full and free, holding endless promise. Over time, however, through repetition, a child hears messages from the adults around him that certain things are not possible or permissible. Slowly the range of allowable experience becomes narrowed by these limits. The child grows into adulthood limited by these accepted ideas.

Affirmation is a process of using repetitive statements to create a desired belief about oneself and life. This process plants the new idea deep within our subconscious mind. In the same way we were programmed as a child we can begin to reprogram ourselves and now exercise choice in the selection of those beliefs.

Using this new found technique of affirmation, Wil began to work on his belief systems. He would start by affirming a willingness to let go of a particular belief that did not serve him. Soon he would add another affirmation alongside the first one. It would be the new belief he now wanted to accept. Over and over he would repeat the process until slowly it was planted like a seed in his subconscious mind.

Gradually he was finding things that before would have caused him to react negatively were loosing their ability to affect him. He was evolving to a new level of experience. He was changing the way he was feeling about life. It was happening not through denying his feelings however. Feelings always need to be expressed. No, he was actually changing his feelings by looking behind them toward the thoughts in his mind from which they emerged. He was now choosing to think differently. This was the one thing he could always have control of. He could choose what to think about the events unfolding in his life. He was beginning to exercise his free will.

BELIEVE IN YOUR DREAMS

Spring was in full bloom and with my new eyes I began to see in unfoldment all around me the propensity toward life inherent within all things. As the small trees along the New York streets awakened from their winter slumber, sending new green leaves stretching toward the sun, the gray city streets of winter began to once more come alive with the colors of spring. In spite of the winter's cruel freeze, the noisy pollution clogged streets and befouled air of the city, the miracle of spring's new birth pressed relentlessly onward. That life could once again come forth from small patches of city ground serving more as latrines for New Yorker's pets than the holy womb of the earth, was a miracle for me.

For the first time I could see in spring's unfoldment the relentless push toward expression in all life. I was beginning to know that I too was no less than the trees and the flowers. From within my own being the new shoots of my true reality were beginning to push through the surface of a seemingly deteriorating body. For the first time the season seemed to affirm back to me the inevitability of my own rebirth. A song began to build in my heart.

There had been a decided change in the way I was coming to view my illness. No longer was it hanging over my head like some ominous breaking storm. Rather, my earlier feelings of complete helplessness were being steadily transformed on a daily basis into a growing awareness that I was able to impact the course of this disease in my body. I could make choices that would alter the course of my life.

The heavy sense of dread that had permeated my entire experience of the last year was giving way to a new sense of hope and excitement. My entire experience with AIDS was slowly shifting in form and was now leading me into hitherto unexplored areas of my self identity. I was increasingly aware I had stepped through an important doorway, even though I was not entirely sure where it would ultimately lead me. I knew, however, I was no longer at a dead end with no way to turn.

My physical condition had also begun to rebound. The tender love and care I was so faithfully lavishing upon my body was finally being returned to me as an increasing feeling of physical well being. I was rebounding quickly from the incapacitating lows of the previous winter. It was not that I was totally symptom free, but where symptoms had been steadily increasing in number, they now ceased to proliferate further. My condition seemed to be stabilizing and my body was showing signs it was capable of dealing with each symptom as it came up.

Spring was in full bloom when my long-time friend Barry Becker suggested I might be interested in reading the Seth material. This series of books had been channeled by Jane Roberts, a trance medium, who spoke for a non-physical entity called Seth. Throughout the 1970's Seth had continued to dictate book after book, using Jane as the channel. These books dealt with the nature of reality as it is experienced by the individual and with the idea that the range of consciousness is much larger than most of us have ever considered possible. These books became my new teachers.

Seth teaches that reality is created for the individual through belief. You believe something is true and it becomes true for you. The limitations that you experience in the body of your life are but reflections of the limited beliefs you hold in your own mind. The only true reality is that you have no limitations, only those you accept through your own belief. When you remove the self-accepted mental barriers, the physical ones then disappear.

These were the most fantastic ideas I had ever encountered! For some people the idea of being responsible for the events of their life is a frightening thought, but for me it was the most hopeful thing I had ever heard. It gave me hope to realize that if I had a hand in creating the illness I was experiencing, then surely I could recreate things another way.

Slowly through my reading I was being shown the role my mind was playing in my individual experience of illness. The Seth material was taking the concept of the Christ mind I had discovered earlier in the Cayce readings, and expanding it. It was then showing me the role I was playing in blocking its expression in my own life. For some, the Cayce material and the Seth teachings are in no way compatible. Cayce's information came from a biblical point of view while Seth's teachings were more scientific in nature. I, however, could see only the commonalities, not the differences. It was on that I chose to focus.

The teachings quickly began to merge together in my mind in such a way that each teaching served to further illuminate the other. I could easily see in my own experience how certain beliefs were limiting my experience. I began to look further at the contents of my own consciousness, seeking to find other limitations I had accepted for myself.

If the Christ mind, one without limitations, was a reality in me, then I was determined to see what beliefs I had accepted that were blocking its expression in my experience. I began to take an inventory of all my beliefs. I looked at what science told me. I looked at medicine. I looked at what religion said. I looked at what my mother told me. I looked at what society said and I looked at what I learned in school. I even looked at Emily Post. Every belief I could find I called into question. If it in any way limited who I was and what I was capable of, I rejected it. I began to write affirmations to deal with the limitations I found in my mind. I began to affirm my safety, my unlimitedness, and my oneness with God. I began the process of slowly re-programming my subconscious mind with my new beliefs in limitlessness. One by one the veils were removed from the eyes of my Christ-self.

My perception of myself and the world around me began

to change and those changes began to accelerate. It was as if the walls in my mind were concentric circles of dominos and as the inner ones were over turned it began a chain reaction outward, opening my mind into the infiniteness of the universal mind.

A growing excitement was building within me as the changes going on in my head rippled out into my day-to-day experience. I could scarcely restrain my impatience in my persistent push toward self-discovery. For now, however, I had gone as far as I could go alone. It was time to reach out for help and support from other people.

In an effort to find the support I needed to continue to unlock the healing power of the mind, I again turned to my good friend Barry Becker. Along with several other interested parties we agreed to form our own study group to further explore the challenges the Seth material presented to us.

In all there were seven of us who began to meet each Wednesday night, that May of 1986. We alternated the gatherings among one another's apartments. There was no set agenda for our meetings. Rather, it became a platform from which each of us could share and then discuss these newly discovered ideas and their application in our daily lives. Each of us had our own reasons for our interest in the material. Although we were all seeking to tap into the deeper psychic levels of the mind, three of us were especially interested in applying what we were learning to our ARC diagnosis.

As we progressed further into the material we began to keep journals of our experiences and to record our dreams. Into our agenda we incorporated group meditations and visualizations on healing, not only for ourselves but for the planet we lived on. What we lacked in understanding we more than made up for in our imagination and enthusiasm for this new way of thinking. We simply made it up as we went along.

Steadily in our own way each of us began to blossom out into different directions, bringing our separate areas of expertise back to the group, enriching one another in countless ways. One by one we began to explore the many avenues of paranormal phenomena available to us.

We investigated and then experimented with the use of crystals as a means of energy amplification and healing. Channeling was also a major source of interest and each one of us explored that phenomena in our own unique way. In time, several members in the group were able to verbally channel their own guides while others of us began receive information delivered through automatic writing. We looked into information on UFOs and extraterrestrials. In whatever directions our individual interests led us we allowed ourselves to pursue. We then brought our discoveries back to the group for their consideration.

The diverse interests of the individuals within the group was a powerful force in expanding the personal range of understanding for each one of us. For me, the group energy served to further accelerate the already considerable progress I had begun on my own. As time passed I found myself more and more attracted to the study of dreams as my personal point of focus. It was upon this exploration I chose to concentrate my efforts during the summer to come.

▲   ▲   ▲   ▲   ▲   ▲   ▲   ▲   ▲   ▲

It was through the instructions laid out in the Seth material that I first began to experiment with my dreams. Although I had always had a vivid dream life, I had never really given much thought to the idea of dream work as a tool for expanding awareness. As I progressed deeper into Seth's writings, however, my desire to begin recording and working with images received in my dreams began to grow.

Using the techniques set forth in the books, before I went to sleep I began to give myself the suggestion that I would remember my dreams. Upon awakening, before I would move from the bed, I would record in a log kept on the night table beside my bed bits of the previous night's dream. I would record just enough to remind me of what I had dreamed and then later I would review the dream and write it as completely as possible in the log. Unless I wrote these random images down immediately upon waking, the memory of the dream would slip away as soon as I left the bed.

Soon I began to recall more than one dream each night, and I would awaken several times a night to record each one. To make things easier I experimented with using a tape recorder. This disturbed Wil from his sleep and so I continued to write them down on paper. I began to experiment with my sleep cycles, dividing them into shorter segments, trying to break down the barriers between my waking and dreaming reality. Soon I advanced to a level where I was able to recognize when I was dreaming and cause myself to become lucid within the dream. In this state I was able to manipulate the dream's outcome.

In a lucid dream one becomes conscious he is dreaming. This happens to most of us naturally in the early morning as we begin to awaken. Sometimes when a dream was enjoyable to me I would deliberately coax it along. Not wanting it to end I found I could literally keep it going while simultaneously being aware it was a dream.

Following the instructions in the Seth material I began to further explore this lucid dream state. I began to find more often than not I could become fully conscious within the dream and could then manipulate the events within it. As I progressed further into this exploration I found that whenever I was experiencing the helpless quality a nightmare engenders, if I were willing to turn and face the event it would change its form. I was then no longer a helpless victim of something beyond my control. Only if I chose to run in fear did the nightmare continue.

One night I had the most incredible out-of-body experience from my dreaming state. Seth had said that if you are dreaming and find yourself in bed but things in your room don't fit what you know to be really there, realize you are dreaming and get out of bed. When you do, you will be out of your body. During a dream one night, I became aware I was dreaming. As I became more lucid within the dream, I realized I was in my bed at home except something was really strange about the room. It was juxtaposed with the work area of my job.

Upon realizing this, a loud voice in my head said to me "Seth says get out of bed". I immediately jumped out of bed. The next thing I knew I was catapulted across my bedroom and flew into the living room. There was a crackling noise inside my head as if it was electrical static on a radio, and I realized I was fully awake and was floating around my living room without my body. I was intensely aware of what was happening to me, that this was no ordinary dream. I was having an out-of-body experience.

As I drifted toward the front door of my apartment I realized I didn't need to open it but could go through it easily. I passed through the door into the hallway and without any real control was sucked down the hall and back into my apartment where I became aware I was under the grand piano in the living room. Slowly I rose up through the piano. I could see the wood inside of the piano and the wires as they passed through my head. It made a sound similar to the scratching of fingernails on a chalk board.

With the piano seemingly passing through the interior of my head, I remember thinking to myself "I had better believe this is possible or Wil may awaken in the morning to find my body mysteriously embedded in the piano." I laughed at the thought.

I then became aware that I was back in the bedroom and was now hovering over my own sleeping form. I could see myself lying on my back and could hear the soft sounds of my own breath as I slept. As I continued to observe my sleeping body a woman who I would later meet in many of my dreams appeared beside me. Looking at my body upon the bed, she turned to me and said "He thinks he's asleep you know". "Yes, I know" I answered, allowing the full realization of this experience to settle in.

Suddenly I was back in my body and I sat up in bed with a start. I was lucid, but still within a dream. Startled, I woke myself up. I lay there for a long time pondering what had happened.

I continued to work with my dreams, recording them and analyzing them for bits of information. As my dream life opened up it spilled forth a rich and expansive reality. So too did my waking life parallel the dreaming one. In every circumstance of my life I was becoming increasingly aware of deeper and deeper dimensions of interactions which I had been asleep to before.

No longer was I just skimming over the surface of my life, but increasingly I was aware of just how inseparable the actor was from the action. I was realizing that the events of my life were not exclusive of me, but were actually changed by my perspective of them. Slowly the intellectual understandings I had gleamed through my studies were becoming heart-felt wisdom. More and more my new beliefs became the platform from which I acted.

By studying my dreams I was coming to a completely new understanding of reality. In a dream, I could experience myself in a location with a body and things seemingly happening to me. The truth was however, I was safe in bed. It was only a hallucination. Instead, I was experiencing my own hopes, fears, beliefs, and dreams acted out in such a way as if they were happening to me. I was literally experiencing my mind from the inside out. Still, I was safe in bed.

By the simple recognition that I was dreaming I was no longer powerless within the dream. Instead, I could take effective action and by facing the nightmare in my mind it was transformed. I was becoming increasingly aware of the countless realities of existence within the realm of human experience. I was also coming to understand the one underlying principle they all held in common. They are all projections of consciousness. They are totally creations of the mind.

I was beginning to see that although in physical reality one deals with time, space, and matter; in truth it is the projection of our beliefs onto the events of life that causes us to experience them in the way we do. In truth these events are neither good nor bad. It is we who give our life the meaning that it has. Through belief we create for ourselves the manner in which our life is experienced.

Incredibly, I was also becoming lucid in the every day nightmare of AIDS that was my conscious experience. I was beginning

to understand that the meanings I was projecting onto the experience of AIDS were causing me to experience it as the death sentence
it was said to be. True, I did have the condition, but I was realizing
I didn't have to accept that the common hysteria around the
experience was the truth about it. Instead, by releasing all my ideas
about the experience and by facing this real life nightmare to see
what it could teach me about myself, I could begin to experience
it in another way. It would begin to change its form.

Ceasing to resist the thing I had feared so much allowed
it to evolve into another experience. By accepting it as simply a
reflection of my own thoughts and feelings AIDS was changing its
form for me. I began to experience it as nothing more than a message
from my body. Through symptoms, my body was seeking to bring
me awareness of things in my own mind about which I was unconscious. I could now choose to use each symptom as a way to
learn about myself.

It was becoming increasingly clear to me that I was not a
victim of a vicious virus that was trying to kill me. Instead, I was
beginning to recognize AIDS as a message from my body. It was
trying to tell me that I was dying from the distorted ideas about
myself I held in my mind. AIDS was my body's attempt to bring
my understanding into a greater alignment with life.

I was not dying of AIDS! Instead, by my limited attitudes
and understandings about life I had been unconsciously committing
suicide all along. AIDS was only making me aware of what I was
doing. It was a loving message from my body. Mistakenly I had
been attacking the messenger instead of responding to the message.
A seemingly impossible shift was occurring in my experience. AIDS
was becoming the greatest teacher about life I had ever encountered.

FORGIVING IT ALL

Spring turned slowly into summer. The one year anniversary of our original diagnosis was approaching. With the bright days of summer there seemed to be an increased clarity about our illness that was coming to replace the bleak days of the previous winter. It was not that suddenly everything in our life was perfect and AIDS was no longer around to be dealt with. It was just that the early feelings of hopelessness and panic were at last receding from our memory to be replaced now with a growing sense of well-being.

No longer was an overwhelming feeling of helplessness steadily gnawing away at my insides. In fact, the ulcer I had given myself from internalized fear upon my diagnosis was fading back into the nothingness from whence it had come. It was now just one more confirmation to me of the power the mind could exert on the physical body. I was almost grateful for its lesson.

The summer season had begun once again on Fire Island. It was a different experience for us both now, however. What had once been a secluded mecca for recreational drug use, free sex, and endless parties, was now a place where we could withdraw into the privacy of our own home. Surrounded by the gentle sounds of the ocean, we spent most of our time alone together except for the occasional company of a close friend. Together we read our books and took long walks on the beach at sunset. I spent a great deal of time planting summer flowers and really noticing for the first time the miraculous intelligence behind their blooming.

After reading "You Can Heal Your Life" by Louise Hay for

the second time, Wil encouraged me to read it again also. Upon first reading we had both found it very Californian, too simple in nature for our New York level of sophistication.

To me it was a simplified version of the Seth material, only it didn't bother to explain how it all worked. Wil, however, had already been convinced through his studies of the mind-body connection of the importance of feelings as the key to health. For him, Louise's teachings about love and forgiveness seemed to be the missing links in his attempts to put himself in a space from which he could avoid reacting so negatively to the things around him. Upon second reading he was so impressed by the book he decided if possible he would like to meet Louise in person. He decided to write to the Hay Foundation in Los Angeles to inquire if she would be in New York City at any time in the near future.

When the door is left ajar, the universe rushes in to fill the need. Only a few hours later that same day as we walked down the boardwalk toward town, there posted on the bulletin board at the harbor was a notice for a Louise Hay seminar. She was scheduled to speak on the upcoming Thursday night and then was to follow it up with a seminar on the weekend. Needless to say when Thursday evening rolled around, Wil and I were two of the first people to show up at the Church that night. We took seats near the front, not wanting to miss a word.

By the time Louise appeared at the podium the church was packed and overflowing. People were standing along the side aisles and across the back of the auditorium. There was a loud buzz of excitement and anticipation as people greeted friends they recognized across the room, surprised to see who among us would be interested in such an approach to AIDS.

At last Louise took to the podium and began to speak. She first told a little about her own personal bout with cancer and then gave some background information on her long interest in metaphysics. She spoke about her belief that disease was a product of mental and emotional toxins, reacting in the body to produce illness. She spoke of the need for self love and acceptance and of the importance of taking 100% responsibility for one's life. It was through taking responsibility for AIDS in one's experience, she said, that one could empower himself to heal it. It could be done through an intense process of personal examination on both a physical and mental level. Forgiveness of the past and of ourself and others was an important key.

I was very excited by Louise's presentation that night. Wil and I had both already come to the place of taking responsibility for our illness. We were sure that it could be healed. We had never before been in the presence of a person, however, who would stand up in a room full of gay people, many of them with AIDS, and many who had lost loved ones near and dear to them, and say we needed to take responsibility for our experience. I was impressed she had the guts to do it and I was excited to see we were not alone in this new understanding about AIDS. Until this time Wil and I had felt very alone in our quest for healing. Now, for the first time, we were in a room packed with other people who were at least open to some extent to these ideas.

At the end, the questions flew hard and fast at Louise. Some people were outraged by her statements. Some people were enthralled. But through it all she stood calmly, fielding every question, never reacting to the turmoil around her. As we left the church that night, Wil and I stopped at the registration tables set up in the back of the room. We signed up for the seminar. It was to be the first seminar either of us had ever attended.

The workshop was to take place on the following Saturday and Sunday and was to run from 9 a.m. until 5 p.m. each day. Each participant was asked to bring a pillow and a stuffed animal with him. Several hundred people showed up and made themselves comfortable on the floor of the hotel ballroom.

The first day of the seminar was filled with many small mental exercises that we accomplished with a partner of our own choosing. Louise would first talk and then after doing an exercise we would spend a great deal of time sharing with the group what had come up for each of us in the exercise. This proved to be one of the most powerful parts of the seminar for me.

Louise passed through the group with the microphone, stopping at each person who wanted to speak. As each person shared bits and pieces of their life, some happy and some so desperate as to make my problems seem insignificant by comparison, we were all drawn toward the realization that our individual pain was shared to some degree by each person in the room that day. I was overwhelmed to discover there was more we had in common with each other than was different about us. I felt drawn out of my isolation into a kinship I had not allowed myself to experience in many years. I was starting to realize I was in no way alone in my experiences. In some way each person in the room was experiencing the same pain.

After completing one of the exercises I was feeling relaxed enough to want to share with the group an insight I had gained from it. I raised my hand and the microphone was brought over to me. Feeling very good about myself for participating so fully, I proceeded to share with the group. When I finished speaking I listened expectantly for Louise's reply, waiting for what I felt would surely be a sign of approval from her. Instead of acknowledging my contribution, she responded to me by pointing out that I had used the word "should" at least seven times while I was sharing. "Should" is a catch-word Louise listens for to make us aware of all the belief programming we operate under. She asked me to just be aware whenever that word came up in my conversation.

I was horrified! Instead of getting approval from this woman who I looked up to, I felt I had been shot down in a most cruel manner. She had done it in front of the entire group. Anger came surging up within me and I was left sitting there by myself to deal with it. I was no longer so sure that this lady was as loving as I had been led to believe. How dare she be so rude to me in front of so many people.

Later during the lunch break I decided I would try once again to establish a better rapport with Louise. Taking my copy of her book, I got in line behind three or four other people who were waiting patiently to speak to her. When it finally came my turn I asked her to autograph my book. When she finished signing, she handed it back to me. I thanked her and went back to my seat to see what she had written. There on the front page were the words "Heal Your Heart, Love Louise".

Again all the anger I had felt before came rushing back to my face. Why was she being so mean to me! How dare she insinuate my heart needed to be healed. My face was twitching as I struggled to deal with my feelings. But dimly in the back of my mind was the awareness that she was right. My heart was the one thing I most needed to heal. It was indeed badly wounded.

At last the first day's session drew to a close. Too exhausted to speak, Wil and I caught a taxi home to get some sleep. We were both emotionally drained by the day's events. We still had another full day of processing to make it through.

During the night Wil awakened to discover he was running a very high fever. His body was aching all over. If this continued through the night, he was not going to be able to go back to the seminar feeling the way he was feeling. Suddenly a light bulb went off in his head. This was an old pattern that he had been using for many years. In the past, whenever he wanted to avoid facing something unpleasant, his body would conveniently create symptoms that would allow him a way out. He was a master at it. On a certain level this was exactly what he was doing now. He wanted to avoid returning to the seminar where he would undoubtedly have to face some unpleasant things about himself.

This time was to be different, however. This time he had a real desire to finally face once and for all these things he had so long avoided. He was not going to allow his body to stop him this time. Instead he began to develop a dialogue with it. He told his body that it might as well cut it out. He was aware of what was going on and it wasn't going to work. He was returning to the seminar the next day even if he was still sick. Finally he drifted back to sleep.

The next morning we both awakened with what felt like

a hangover. Wil's fever was long gone. I, on the other hand, didn't want to get out of bed and my chest felt constricted by a great sadness. All of the emotions that had been stirred up by the previous day seemed to be stuck now in my throat. I climbed out of bed and began to iron a shirt to wear. Suddenly I burst into tears. I didn't want to go back and spend another day with that woman. I didn't want to put myself through any more pain. Wil wouldn't let me back out and he insisted we finish the seminar. We returned to the hotel for the second session.

All during the second day of the seminar I was feeling a great sadness. Whenever someone in the crowd would share something sad or painful, the tears would instantly well up in my eyes. My heart was resonating in empathy as time after time I heard my own pain expressed through the words of other people. I remained quietly withdrawn the entire day, however, not willing to risk sharing again. I just allowed myself to feel whatever was happening in my heart.

For almost the entire day we dealt with issues revolving around our childhood and family. It became obvious that the ideal family we all held in our mind was just a myth, one of many we had been led to believe in. No one there seemed to have had a childhood in any way resembling it. Instead most of us were getting in touch with how much we needed to forgive various members of our family.

As a closing exercise, Louise chose one dealing with forgiveness. We were each to choose a partner. Sitting cross-legged on the floor, holding hands and looking each other in the eye, one was to say to the other, "I forgive you ____ for ____ ." The other person was to reply "Thank you, I set you free".

Since I had chosen strangers as partners all day, I chose Wil to do this final exercise with me. As I said the words, my father's name came up to fill in the blank. As I continued to finish the statement I said, "I forgive you for not loving me when I was a child." Before I could finish the sentence, a great heaving sob rolled out of my chest and I began to cry uncontrollably. The pain I had felt for more than 30 years around my relationship with my father, came pouring out of me in great waves. I continued to cry until finally there were no more tears to shed.

Wil held me in his arms as I just laid there exhausted and unable to move. I felt as though a huge weight had been lifted from my shoulders. There was a light ringing in my ears. As I rose to my feet it was as if I were walking two feet off the ground.

This was the power of forgiveness! In those few tearful moments I had released an incredible load of pain I had been holding inside myself since childhood. In the clarity of mind which that release brought, I realized for the first time the part I had played in that drama. It was I who had withdrawn my love from my father, not the other way around. I had projected all the judgments I had learned from my religious upbringing onto him. Because I judged him to be everything one ought not to be, I had cut off my love from him. His love for me had always been there. It was I who was unable to accept it.

In that moment of forgiveness an entire chapter of my past was completely rewritten. An experience I had believed to be true for over thirty years, in an instant was transformed. In its place came the realization that in truth it had never happened as I remembered. There was no one to forgive except myself. I could literally feel the physical effect the release of that judgment created in my body. All the energy, that until now had been used to nurse my resentment, was now free to flow through my body. I could hardly keep my balance as it rushed through me. As the seminar came to an end, I floated home a happy but exhausted man.

Louise Hay's work brought more pieces of the puzzle of healing to me. I began to fully realize just how important forgiveness is as a way of releasing one's self from the past in order to live fully once again without judgment in the present.

For years I had, through unforgiveness, allowed my resentments about my childhood to affect the way in which I dealt with my present life. It had colored my self-esteem and actions in every relationship I had formed since my childhood. It had consumed massive amounts of my life energy, using it to nurse the pain and resentment I held. Now forgiveness had set me free to experience things in a new way. It was allowing me to live in the present moment, no longer haunted by the events of the past.

I was also beginning to feel at a deep level what it means to be one with all life. The seminar showed me that beneath all the superficial personality differences, we are all so very much alike. In our own individual ways we yearn for the same things. We all hurt for the same reasons.

I was learning through my own suffering to feel compassion for others. My most basic perceptions of myself and my relationship to others was rapidly being transformed. I was coming to understand I was not alone and I became increasingly willing to reach out to others.

In the weeks following the workshop, I sought to apply the lesson of forgiveness to every experience of my life. I searched through my mind for distant memories of hurts I had long since pushed down and aside, but had never really faced and released. Through my childhood memories I searched for any slight I could remember, and when I found one I called it forward to be examined closely and then forgave it all- myself included. For me it no longer had anything to do with who was right or wrong. It had only to do with setting my own self free.

As I sought to forgive my past, my perceptions of those events became enlarged to include both sides of the picture. I was more aware than I had ever been of how I had unconsciously cooperated in the formation of those events. This awareness was an outgrowth of the increasing responsibility I was taking in my own present life and healing. As I released my judgment of past events, new memories of happy times long since forgotten came back into remembrance once again. The entire memory of my childhood began to shift and change, taking on a softness where once the edges had been rough.

I continued to extend forgiveness into the everyday events of my life. Using Louise's tapes each evening I would forgive and release the events of the day. Consistently I continued to practice forgiveness until I was increasingly able to extend it in each and every moment. I was evolving toward the point in my own consciousness where judgment and forgiveness were merging together into total acceptance in each present moment. This was a vantage point from which I had never before experienced reality and it was becoming increasingly clear to me it was the only place I wanted to be.

For Wil the seminar had served to confirm for him once again how necessary it was to put himself in a space of feeling love. It had also given him the piece to the puzzle he had been missing until now, the tool that would transform his stress into ease. This tool was forgiveness. He did not need to know how it worked, he only had to be willing to forgive.

For Wil there was a situation with a co-worker that seemed to him to be an ideal opportunity to demonstrate that love and forgiveness would really work. He felt if he could forgive this particular woman then he could be sure he could forgive anyone. If this situation could be transformed, then anything could be.

Several months earlier, shortly after Wil's diagnosis with KS during a period where I was home in bed very sick, Wil had gotten into a tremendous fight with this supervisor. After working overtime for several days to finish up some year end reports, Wil had slipped out for a couple of hours in order to run home and check on how I was doing. As soon as he left work, his supervisor came in and discovered that he was not in the office. By the time he arrived home to check on me, the phone was already ringing.

A tremendous fight ensued. All of the pent-up anxiety and frustration he had been holding for months burst loose. The argument degenerated until both Wil and his supervisor were cursing at one another. In the end they swore never to work together again. Since that day there had been an icy coldness between them. Each went out of his way to avoid contact with the other.

Wil felt if he had ever hated anyone, then this woman was the one. Now he was facing the realization that his anger at her was only hurting him. It was just one more thing suppressing his immune system. For his own sake, he knew he was going to have to forgive her.

Using a visualization process from Louise Hay's book, Wil began to do daily forgiveness work on the woman. First he would put her on a stage. With his imagination he would see the most horrible things he could imagine happening to her. He would see her jobless and humiliated. He would see her being ripped to shreds by wild animals. When finally his anger was entirely spent, he would see her on stage once again. This time she would have all the things in life she desired given to her. He would see her feeling fulfilled and happy. Then, after this was finished, it was his turn on stage, having all the deep wishes of his heart come true. He would see himself healthy and complete. He continued to do this on a daily basis until his anger slowly began to subside.

After a few weeks he began to notice that on occasion, while passing in the hall, their eyes would meet for a brief moment without looking away. And soon thereafter their passing would elicit a brief nod and sometimes a slight smile. Before long they were even beginning to have some superficial conversation, when on occasion they would meet at the coffee wagon.

One day while walking down the hall, the supervisor called Wil into her office. After asking him to take a seat, she told him there was something she needed to share with him. "For the last two months I have been sending you love," she told him. Wil almost fell out of the chair! By some impossible coincidence they had both been doing the same thing to each other. They could scarcely believe it.

As their individual stories tumbled out they discovered they had both been under a tremendous amount of stress at the time of their fight. A good friend of hers had just died of AIDS at the same time Wil was having to deal with his own diagnosis. They both had used a slight misunderstanding as a convenient outlet for venting all their bottled up frustrations on each other. They had been the perfect mirrors for one another.

As the weeks passed a friendship between the two of them began to grow. They continued to share with one another the personal events of their separate lives and the trials and tribulations of beginning a spiritual path. Within short period of time they had become the closest of friends.

This experience became another turning point in Wil's healing. Here he had experienced the overwhelming power of love and forgiveness on a first hand basis. He had seen what to him had seemed an impossible situation, transformed into a beautiful and lasting friendship.

Slowly the intellectual understandings he had gleaned from medical research were being transformed into emotional realities. The ideas that had once only floated in his head without any real tangibility were becoming the reality of his everyday experience. The work of love and forgiveness was at last moving him out of his head and into his heart. He was beginning to really feel his feelings. Before he had only thought them. His commitment to his new found beliefs was deepening.

THE DREAM IS REALIZED

As June pressed on into July, I again renewed my commitment to my dream work. It was not that I had been able to get answers to all my problems through recording and interpreting my dreams. It was just that as time went on, an awareness was growing within me of the broader implications of the things I had experienced through analyzing the dream reality.

There had been lucid dreams and dreams in which I was able to go out of my body. I had been able to enter fully conscious into my own dreams and to manipulate their outcome. I had done things that a short time before I would have doubted possible.

Long before this time, I had recognized the fact that AIDS had all the qualities of a nightmare. No matter how one tried to escape it, everything was set up to tell you there was no way out. Every step taken in the direction of self-empowerment seemed to be negated by lapses into helplessness. Always, the virus was lurking in your body, just waiting for the right time to do you in.

Now as I began , one by one, to let go of the beliefs I held that were limiting me in any way, I began to experience myself differently. I had long ago accepted the truth of my identity and to the best of my abilities I had sought through prayer and meditation to bring more of that realization into manifestation in my life. Through the everyday events of my own life, I was purposefully seeking to apply the new beliefs I had accepted. I scrutinized the mirror my life afforded, looking for clues to the blockages in my own mind. And through my dream work I had begun to explore dimensions of my consciousness beyond just the narrow physical experience.

How my life was changing! I was at last beginning to step out of the many boxes I had put myself in. My deepest desire had become to know myself in the truest spiritual sense. What had started in fear as a search for physical healing, had somehow become a search for myself in spiritual terms.

I now knew beyond a shadow of a doubt that the healing I was seeking would come only as a result of finding this spiritual connection. I committed with all my heart to remove all the self-imposed blockages in consciousness preventing me from the realization of my true nature. I was sure the physical healing would occur naturally as a result.

I knew that for me, the illness was not about the germs and viruses. By now I knew they were not the true cause of my illness. AIDS was about the distortions in my own perception of which my illness was the result. In six short months I had almost completely freed myself of Western medicine's limited perception of health and dis-ease. I had seen past these man-made belief systems to the deeper truth of my condition. It had been made easy for me. By offering me nothing, medicine had forced me to rely upon my own innate resources. It was these resources that had brought me through to this point.

It was through a dream that I came into awareness of my own healing. There is no way to accurately describe what happened to me in that moment, yet in an instant my belief in the possibility of my own healing was transformed into the knowledge that it was done.

I was floating through space. I seemed to be supported on all sides as one might be when floating upon a warm salty sea. A blinding flash of white light surrounded me and flowed through every atom of my body. A wave of ecstasy, as in an orgasm, coursed through my body and I felt a tingle of electricity in each and every cell. I was engulfed by feelings of immense love and protection as I floated on effortlessly, suspended in this white light. These feelings continued to break upon me in endless waves.

I awakened from my sleep, lying quietly in my bed. I could still feel the sensations of the dream throughout my body. For a moment I believed it was some kind of sexual dream and I touched myself, seeking to find an emission. There was none. I laid very still and allowed the feelings to continue through me. I knew something incredible had occurred, something I had never before experienced. The feelings of warmth and safety continued to pour over me. I began to cry softly.

I lay there that night for at least an hour, basking in the divine love that was flowing through me, until at last I drifted off to sleep once again. When I woke the next morning I was still carrying those incredible feelings with me. I was almost afraid to allow myself the realization now growing in my heart. For three days I carried the memory of the dream with me until at last the realization burst fully into my consciousness. I had touched that place deep within me where the reality of my wholeness had remained forever untouched. And from that place would wholeness now manifest into my physical body, its path unblocked by any remaining obstructions.

I told Wil that night about my dream experience. I told him I would no longer continue to take the medicines I had sought so hard to acquire in Mexico. There was no longer a need for medicine to kill the virus. The virus was not really the enemy. There was no enemy without, only the thoughts and feelings within me that had served to undermine my God given sovereignty. The walls and defenses I had built around myself that kept love out were the only real enemies I had. They were the result of a belief in my own lack of safety; a basic failure to recognize myself for who I truly am. I had built defenses in the belief they protected me and made me strong. In reality they were only reflections of a belief in my own weakness.

When one is strong, he needs no walls for protection. Peace through might is a deception of the ego mind. He who wields force is weak. Only in the laying down of all defense is true strength recognized.

AIDS is complete biological vulnerability. In my own experience, it was reflecting back to me in the condition of my physical body, the belief behind all the defenses I had erected between myself and others. It was a belief in my total vulnerability.

And now the healing had come, not from killing some hostile virus. It had come in the piece by piece dismantling of all the thought systems and defenses I had so carefully constructed to hide behind. My strength had returned from laying my weapons down. I was no longer able to think of myself in terms of illness. In my own mind I knew the healing I had sought was accomplished.

In my months of reading metaphysical teachings I had become sure of one thing. There is nothing existing in this physical world that did not exist first in someone's mind. It was first a thought or a vision and then, unless fear or limitation were allowed to block the process, it would at last emerge as a physical reality. I knew in that moment of dreaming that my healing was real in my mind and heart. I had spent the last six months of my life removing any blocks that would keep it from being my reality. Physical healing was now only a matter of time.

Wil was afraid for me to discontinue the medicine. He did not fully understand what I was telling him, and was afraid I was deluding myself into believing what I desperately wanted to be true. After all, there was as yet no apparent change in my physical condition and we both knew my T-cells were severely depressed. There was no way for me to fully explain to him what had occurred. There was no experience in my life I could relate it to in an effort to explain it to him. I just knew I was well.

In the months that followed, the healing that had occurred instantaneously on the level of spirit, began to be made manifest throughout my physical body. Slowly, my body became aware of what my heart already knew. My blood test results reversed direction and began an ascent back towards the range of normal.

Each day my body responded to the increased energy flow of life force energy through it. Every inner wall that fell sent a greater flow of life force energy coursing through it. My heart literally began to sing within my chest. Every new day burst upon me with more life and joy than I had ever experienced before. I saw things through new eyes of gratitude. It was so incredible to me that a homosexual hairdresser living in the fast lane in New York City could, through AIDS, come to know himself as a beloved son of God. I laughed at the unlikeliness of it all!

With each passing day I continued to stretch my heart open just a little further, and tried just a little harder to see beyond the surface of things to the truth that lies within. My judgments of life continued to fall away and an increasing allowance came to take its place. I began to see beauty in places where it had never existed for me before. This just served to drive me further along. I knew that the beauty I was now seeing all around me was nothing less than a reflection of my own.

▲   ▲   ▲   ▲   ▲   ▲   ▲   ▲   ▲   ▲

After the seminar in June, Wil's experiences with love and forgiveness had only served to strengthen his commitment to extend it throughout his entire life experience. He began a daily practice of sending love to whatever person or event that would enter his mind. He found the fifteen minutes a day he spent riding the subway to work was basically wasted time. He began to fill that time with many different mental exercises.

He was coming to view every experience in his life as an opportunity to express love. It did not matter if it were in a taxicab with the driver, a restaurant with a waiter, or in a board meeting at work. The form of the encounter was really not what was important, only the opportunity to experience love with another person.

Increasingly his experience was reflecting back to him his loving intent. Even the roughest edges of his life had begun to soften and smooth under his commitment to love. More than anything, love was putting him in a space from which people could react to him in a different way. No more was he coming from a defensive space of caution that so often in the past had drawn attack to him. His new openness was being reflected back to him by the loving responses of others.

He was certain that love also had physiological ramifications. The opening of his heart had a direct effect on his thymus gland. Here was where the T-4 cells of his body matured. Even his chronic colitis problem that had defied all medical attempts to solve it, had begun to ebb. Love had replaced the knot in his stomach with a warm glow in his chest.

Wil had also begun the practice of visualization. He had come an incredible distance from that recent point in the past when he had scoffed at the very same idea. Now he found himself spending nearly a half-hour each day exploring creative ways to visualize his healthy blood cells attacking and killing the virus. He found it was one area in which he could allow his full creativity to flow without feeling self-conscious. There was no one there to judge him, just himself with his imagination. He was proving to be very skillful in its use.

More and more however, there seemed to be one aspect of his visualization that bothered him. In all other aspects of his life he was trying to extend and experience love. Yet he would come home at the end of the day and wage a war against the virus. He would turn his body into a battleground. It was a paradox that had not failed to gain his attention.

After giving it considerable thought, he came to the decision there was only one way around this dilemma. Although he had never heard of anyone else doing such a thing, he decided he would have to change the very nature of his visualizations. Instead of continuing to attack and kill the virus, he began to visualize an energy of love coming into his body through the top of his head. This energy spread slowly throughout his body and down into his legs where the lesions were. Gently he began to stroke the lesions with this energy, caressing them softly. He visualized this love energy totally enveloping the virus. He then began talking to it softly. He reassured it that it was in a safe and loving body. It was so safe in fact, it could feel free to go to sleep if it wanted to.

Within a matter of a few weeks he began to notice some of the lesions on his legs seemed to be getting lighter. It was almost imperceptible at first, maybe nothing more than an overactive imagination. Encouraged, he continued to visualize religiously, paying careful attention to the color of the lesions. Soon there was no doubt they were getting lighter. He could hardly believe his eyes.

It was during this time I came to Wil with my decision to discontinue taking the medications we had obtained in Mexico. At first this caused him to experience a great deal of fear. Although he was taking on new beliefs about healing, in the back of his mind was still the thought that it was the medication that was going to do the job. All of these other ideas were helpful on a certain level, but there was still a lingering belief in a magic pill. This was a belief system he had held for over forty years. It could not be let go of overnight.

As he thought about it further, however, he had to admit there really was no guarantee the medicine was of any real value to begin with. Besides, he could hardly argue with what was becoming more obvious with each passing day. My physical condition was visibly improving. There was a smile on my face and a light in my eyes that was even brighter than the days before either one of us had ever heard of AIDS. There certainly was no doubt I was getting better. He began to think perhaps he needed to incorporate more of my techniques into his own healing path.

Shortly, Wil was to arrive at his own fork in the road where he too would decide whether to continue with the medication or not. By this time however, he had let go of some of the initial fears he had experienced upon learning I had made the decision to quit taking my medicine. He could see that my health had not suddenly fallen apart. Now he was faced with the same decision, but for different reasons. His reasons were more pragmatic in nature. For him, the worsening side effects, among them severe anemia, were beginning to outweigh any of the perceived benefits. More and more he was encountering information that cast a cloud of doubt over whether these medications had any real benefits at all. He was growing increasingly concerned that the toxic effects of the medication would jeopardize the progress he was beginning to make on other fronts. Before long, he too discontinued their use.

Upon my suggestion, Wil finally began to entertain the idea of meditation. It was the one thing he had been avoiding from the very beginning. For him it had too many spiritual connotations and spirituality had never been a subject that was very near and dear to his heart. And yet he wanted to find the answers he needed for the healing. But sometimes it seemed to him the answers always lay where he wished they didn't. If he was sincerely seeking the truth, however, it would have to be accepted where it was found, not only where he wished it to be.

Being a good programmer and being used to working with a manual, he went to the bookstore and purchased a "how to" book on meditation. After reading the book he went into the living room, put on soft music, lowered the lights, and promptly fell asleep. Those times he did manage to stay awake, his mind raced so fast there seemed no possible way to quiet it down. But he kept with it, and before long found the doorway into his inner reality and crossed the threshold within.

It was deep within in meditation that he first encountered the awareness of a divine intelligence permeating all of existence. And slowly the recognition grew that this same intelligence was expressing itself as the life-force through his own body; that he was a unique example of this intelligence in expression. And so was this same intelligence expressing through each and every living thing in existence. Slowly the relationship of all life to each of its parts revealed itself to him. With that came the understanding that as you do to another, you have done to yourself. On a deeper level of being that other person you judge is you. He came to realize that by sending love to others he had actually been sending love to himself.

He began to go to the teacher within through meditation and asked the questions whose need for answers had become so clear. "How is this illness serving me?" "How can I face this situation and learn from it?" "What are the changes this experience is seeking to bring me?" "What is this allowing me to do that I didn't do before?"

As he grew in willingness to relate each experience back to himself, so too were the understandings of each situation increasingly revealed on ever deeper levels. He found a profound shift occurring in his experience with the illness. No longer did it seem that he was dying from an incurable illness. Rather with the acceptance of each new symptom as a communication from his body, the illness was taking on the nature of an accelerated course in living. Instead of moving deeper into the illness, with each new symptom he was being propelled forward at an amazing rate of speed.

His body was purging itself with each new symptom. As he faced each one willingly, it was quickly released, elevating him to a greater awareness of life.

He was no longer dying of AIDS. He was healing into life through the experience of the disease. It was a profound difference in understanding of what to an outside observer would have appeared to be a continuation of symptoms. But more clearly in his mind each day was the knowledge that he was headed in a new direction. A day would come when there would be no symptoms for his body to release.

As the shift continued it became increasingly clear there was a growing conflict between his new awareness of his condition on a personal level, and what was being reflected back to him in his interactions with the traditional medical establishment. Any feelings he had that he might be experiencing his illness as anything other than an endless downward spiral, were totally invalidated each time he received the results of his medical test.

The T-Cell test in particular was one that over and over served to negate his emerging thoughts of healing. The power these numbers now held, not only over him, but over every person with a positive antibody test result, was enormous. The general public had attached tremendous meaning to the outcome of these numbers which, until AIDS, had literally been unheard of. He had even known of people who had considered suicide upon learning of a particularly low count.

He knew he needed to quit attaching so much meaning to the test. Most doctors themselves, when pressed closely, would reluctantly admit that even they were unclear as to the number's real importance. There were even studies to suggest that the normal range of fluctuation could be very large indeed. Still, there were many people with AIDS who decided whether to get up or stay in bed for the day as a result of their T-cell count.

Wil made an agreement with himself. He no longer wanted to know the result of his T-cell test. Whether they went up or down he had found made little difference. His mind could use even an improvement as a way of beating him up. If the counts did improve, it was never enough. He decided, for his own sake, he no longer wanted to know.

If the doctor needed the numbers for his own information, then Wil would submit to the test. But the doctor could keep the results to himself. He could be the one to worry about the numbers, and if he felt some new therapy were in order he could suggest it. Wil's end of the bargain would be as follows: each day on arising from bed he would meditate. In meditation he would ask himself this question. "If my T-cell count were to go down today, what would I do now that I have not been doing before?" And whatever came up for him, he would do it. He would not wait for a negative test result to scare him into taking action. He would just do, on a daily basis, everything within his power to create health and happiness in his life.

As time passed, the decision to let go of the test results began to pay off. No longer were they always there to throw a blanket of doubt and fear over the hope building daily within his heart. And that hope was in turn reacting within his physical body to create an environment in which healthy functioning could return to his immune system.

His efforts to experience love had by this time rippled out to touch each and every sector of his life. Even his virus and the lesions on his legs had been included within that love. They were responding in turn by becoming more friend than foe. There had been no further progression of Kaposi Sarcoma on his body. It was not continuing to follow what was by now the expected inevitable progression. It had been halted completely, and what lesions remained were slowly being reabsorbed into his body.

The visits to the doctor, which had for so long been on a weekly basis, were growing to be less frequent now. The seemingly unending stream of annoying infections, both real and imagined, was slowing to a halt. And when periodically a symptom would arise, it was greeted by a different perception. Just one more message from the body, another fine tuning of his consciousness. It was now a new consciousness, completely transformed and expanded into a greater alignment with life by each symptom that had been faced for its message and lovingly released when the lesson was learned.

BEYOND AIDS

Time was passing more quickly now. The long days of summer had long since given way to the brisk coolness of fall. A touch of winter was in the air. 1987 was just around the corner. We were back in the city now, swept up in the relentless pace of living there. But beyond this flurry of activity, at the center of our lives, was a sense of calm, clear detachment from it all. It was truly a safe place from which to weather even the most fierce of storms. From this place it seemed nothing outside could possibly shatter our calm. There was nothing out there that would not yield to that peace.

For each of us, the time was fast approaching when the need to learn through symptoms would no longer be necessary. The old thought patterns and feelings of guilt and fear, that at one time had poisoned our minds and rippled out into our experience to distort our lives and health, had been lovingly faced and long since erased from our consciousness. In their place was a new understanding, born in response to that experience. It was the knowledge of who we are, valued players in the greater cosmic scheme of creation.

Our lives, which before had seemed but a desperate grab for a moments' fleeting joy in the face of a world designed to snatch it all away, had been transformed in stature to a gift. It was a gift with purpose and meaning, far beyond the mundane realities of social consciousness. Step-by-step, our minds had been set free. We had broken loose from a man-made prison of limiting belief. We had been liberated into the freedom that comes only in knowing the intelligence behind all things lives within each one of us.

With each new day, an increasing vitality was returning to Wil's body. With persistent visualization, his lesions had continued to fade until finally they were no longer visible at all. His T-cells, once numbering below one hundred, were once again within the range of normal. His immunological profile was becoming such that it no longer revealed this was a person with AIDS. The doctor visits, once so frequent in nature, were now only once every several months. Now they were just for the purpose of allowing the doctor to see how well he was doing and to document the results.

Unlike mine, his healing had not come with the dramatic realization of a dream. Rather it had blossomed slowly as a seed of hope, planted in the fertile ground of a mind willing to embrace the impossible. It had been watered and fed and tendered until now in its logical conclusion it had burst forth as a flower into bloom.

It had not been necessary to force the petals open. It had been nothing more than the gentle allowance of a natural process, left to its inevitable conclusion. Like a gardener, all that could be done had been done. Yet there was the understanding that the process of life was accomplished by a power far greater than the gardener himself.

This was the paradox of healing. The outcome was made possible through surrender. To do everything within one's power and yet to relinquish the result. How difficult was this lesson in a world where the belief is that the only thing that truly matters is the result. And yet only by detachment from the result can it be truly owned.

Like a butterfly emerging from a cocoon, so too did Wil take a final step out of a rigid sense of self-identity into the truth of his limitless reality. The constraining vice of an intellect directed by the judgments of the ego was liberated into the knowledge of the heart. His physical appearance began to change. His face rounded and softened and became younger in appearance. His style of dressing, once only shades of black and gray, blossomed with the colors of a peacock's feathers. All the while, I just watched and smiled with joy to see the physical unfoldment of a mind set fully free.

In my own life the internal changes continued to transform my experience. In every area of my life, my new beliefs were rippling out from my center to bring change to everything they touched. My attitude toward life took on the element of trust.

It was not that I never again experienced fear. Nor was it that suddenly my life became perfection. It was just that now I no longer ran away from the things I feared. For now I had tools I never had before. And I knew going into the fear was exactly where I needed to go. Now I could use my fear for growth. The thing I most wanted to avoid was the place I would now go freely. Through the willingness to face each fear, I was inevitably propelled beyond it, onto a new plateau of life, a slightly higher elevation from which I could see just a little more of the total picture of my life.

I was achieving perfection in the only area of my life where perfection was possible. I was becoming perfect in my willingness to take responsibility for everything occurring in my life. I would no longer place blame outside myself. And no longer would I cripple myself, agonizing over another's role in anything I experienced. The only thing important to me now were my reasons for my own reactions to those events.

No longer did I ask, "Why did I create this?" every time something happened in my life I didn't particularly care for. Instead the question had now become "How can I respond to this right now in such a way that I experience growth from it?" And as I asked "How", very shortly the "Why" would reveal itself to me, a by-product of my willingness to forgive in each moment.

That is what the physical healing had been also. It had been a by-product of my quest to heal my heart and mind. To be sure, I had done many things on a physical level. I had detoxified my body and explored nutrition. I had given up cigarettes and drugs. I had begun to exercise, have massages, and see a chiropractor. But each one of these things I had done only as a result of first changing my mind. Then the physical things followed as a natural result of those changes.

In a little over a year and a half I had emerged from a seemingly impenetrable darkness into a new life. Every cell of my being had been dismantled piece by piece, and my reality had been reconstructed from the ground up. My outlook on myself and life had been completely transformed.

My understanding of the role of illness within the process of life had been drastically altered. It was only a road to a greater awareness of living. Through my simple willingness I had been able to see beyond the outer appearance of AIDS in my life to the gift within it. I had come to understand the only sure thing in life was that every experience has a gift to give. And only in a willingness to see beyond the outer wrappings can it be received.

How much easier to respond to the message than to kill the messenger. This was the beauty of truth, it was simple. It was not always easy to face in the panic of the moment, but always it was simple. Like clouds before the sun, appearances could obscure but never change reality. Of this I was sure.

As my focus changed, the picture of my life took on new details. People I had considered real friends were suddenly nowhere to be found. And some people I would have never expected it of, drew closer. At work, within my clientele, there was a change as one-by-one I began to share with each one my experience with AIDS. I began first with the ones I knew I could trust and told them. Then I began to tell the others. Until finally everyone knew. Some of them never returned again. Others did. But I did not care. No longer could I hide the truth about myself in fear I would lose their love and support. I knew what hiding had done to me before. I would never do that to myself again. Gone was the crazy belief I could get love by hiding what I felt was unlovable about myself.

As some people chose to leave my life, so too did others come to fill the gaps their leaving caused. I hid nothing from these new people. And for this they seem to love me. Each willingness on my part to be honest about myself released a little more life-force energy into my body. For every secret exposed, a greater freedom came to take its place.

No more would I contract around my fear, holding it deep within me. Instead, I chose to breathe into the pain, creating an opening through which it could be released. There was no longer anything to hide, nothing left to fear. Just a growing sense deep within me of what it truly means to be free.

PART II
Expanded
Perceptions

▲ TOWARD A NEW UNDERSTANDING

Of all the distorted perceptions we experience in our lives, the one that lies at the root of all the many others is the misconception of who we really are and what, if any, purpose or meaning our lives entail. In our 20th Century, science and technology have contributed greatly to many misconceptions about life by isolating us from the natural world, where we could more clearly see and understand the realities of life and our relationship to the larger world as a whole.

As we huddle together in our large urban centers, we insulate ourselves from the natural world by our many structures, both physical and psychological. We block out the sky, the dawn, and the sunset, and then lose ourselves in our man made realities. If we will allow it, however, all roads lead home. Even through our physical sciences we can learn the greater truths of life.

When our scientists and physicists peer through their electron microscopes in search of the most minute particles which are the building blocks of the material world, what they find, to their astonishment, is that the electrons circulating around the nucleus of an atom express themselves in two ways - either as a particle or as an energy wave. In the reality of the microcosmic world of subatomic particles, there is no basic building block of matter. Rather, there is a tendency for energy that is in constant motion to manifest as a particle.

The physical world we experience, the matter composing

the objects we take for granted as being solid and real, is in reality pure energy slowed until it manifests in a denser form - matter. The truth of this material universe in which we live is, if we had eyes and could perceive in a broader range of frequencies, we would see our precious physical world as pulsating flows of energy, constantly moving and continuously vibrating!

Behind this pulsating energy, there is an intelligence that builds it into the patterns from which all the objects of our physical world are formed. It is the intelligence that causes the seed to achieve its potential as a flower, a caterpillar to undergo a metamorphosis, emerging as a butterfly, and an embryo to grow into a perfectly formed baby. It hangs the stars in space into their perfect orbits. This intelligence and the energy on which it acts, the very matter out of which we all are formed, is what we have come to know as God - totality of thought and being, ALL THAT IS. This force, the very life-force itself, is creative love. This same force seeks to operate in our lives if we will allow it.

One of the disservices of modern science is to put forth the belief that the universe was formed by accident, that life came about as the result of an accidental mixing of the primeval soup, and therefore has no purpose or meaning. This belief gave rise to an age of fatalism, the belief in luck and chance. We have been brought up to believe we are acted upon by forces outside ourselves over which we have no control. Our lack of conscious knowledge of life's purpose and meaning has caused our experiences to reflect this ignorance.

The truth is that God is everywhere present, omniscient, and omnipotent. We exist in and are made of ever-present creative love. We exist in a medium which ceaselessly seeks to propel us toward our greatest unfoldment. The same creative love that pulls the acorn toward expression as an oak is in operation in our lives. And yet through our lack of awareness, it has little effect on us.

When we look through a microscope at the configuration of an atom, we can see the nucleus, surrounded by electrons and protons. And through a telescope we observe the planets, with their moons and satellites in orbit around them, the solar system with her sun and the planets encircling it, and on into the galaxies, themselves spinning around a distant center. Through observation we can see a property of the universe holding true for all of her creations. This property is that knowledge of the whole is inherent within the smallest particle. Our sciences are just now discovering this truth in their attempts at the process of cloning. From the DNA information in a single cell is the knowledge to create from that one cell the complete structure from which it is taken.

On this physical plane, man is the creative intelligence. Inherent within him is the knowledge of his greater potential, the God within. We as homosapiens are the physical vehicle by which the creative intelligence behind all things seeks to explore its own creation. Our human body is but the developing embryo that is to become the vehicle through which divine mind seeks to clothe itself in physical form.

We use only 10% of the capacity of our brains, the rest lies dormant, seemingly beyond reach. In the genius we glimpse the potential within each of us. Still, we feel it is the exception to the norm. Genius is the birthright of each and every one of us. It is the limited experience we accept as the norm that is the aberration. Because of our beliefs we do not allow ourselves knowledge of our true self, the God within. Instead, we accept an impostor identity, the ego, altered by belief in limitation, as our true self. The divine within becomes an unrealized dream.

We have lost faith in the purpose and meaning of our lives. Without faith, real growth and healing are not possible. When there is no growth, there is stagnation and death. This is what we as a species are facing unless we begin to expand beyond our current definitions of who we are.

Faith is an aspect of consciousness. Whether we have faith in God or in nothing, that is what we will draw into our experience. Faith is the power of our own belief. Our fears are simply misplaced faith. When faith is put in things outside of oneself, whether science or technology, fame or fortune, to that extent we have negated the power within us. When the outer things no longer have an answer for us, then we have nothing on which to rely. Our gods are found to have feet of clay.

The only thing that can not be taken away is the God-Self that lies within. When faith is applied to the answers coming from within the heart, this faith can never fail us. For we have put ourselves in the hands of a universal intelligence in which there is no possibility of failure.

Through faith in the God within, dependence on the answers of our own heart, we gain independence from the outer effects of the world - disease and lack. To the degree we look outside of ourselves for answers, to that degree have we given our freedom away. We must shift our focus inwardly, relying on the communications of the heart. There is the seat of wisdom, our connection to a greater knowing that will lead us home.

REALITY

In the dream state, one experiences a reality that is a construction of the mind. Although we experience ourselves there with a body and in seemingly concrete surroundings, it is totally a construction of our mind. In the dream state we meet the contents of our conscious minds in an elaborate three dimensional production. Our fears and possibilities are acted out in such a way that we experience them outside of ourselves, as if they were happening to us.

We can run from the monsters in our nightmares, but they will always continue to chase us. In reality they are a projection of our own unconscious fears. To end the nightmare, we must not slay the dragon out there, but instead turn inward, to examine the fears we hold in consciousness which are its source.

Almost each and every one of us has experienced a lucid dream. In a lucid dream we become conscious we are dreaming. If the dream is pleasant we can extend it at will, consciously directing its course. If it is a nightmare we can wake ourselves up to the reality that we are in the safety of our bed.

The physical reality we accept as concrete is but one perception of the countless realities occurring simultaneously. In physical reality the root assumptions of time and space are different than in the dream state where time is non-sequential and distance is not experienced. The underlying truth, however, is that all reality is a construction of the mind.

In objective physical reality we meet the contents of our mind in the out-picturing of our own bodies and the circumstances of our lives. It is presented to us in a three-dimensional form of fantastic intricacy. Everywhere we turn we see reflected back to us our own self. The world we live in is formed out of the objectified contents of our mind.

It is the purpose of life to know oneself completely. By this mental projection mechanism we are given the opportunity to meet our thoughts about ourselves and our relationship to others as the circumstances of our life. Through this experience we can learn the truth of our being. The reality we experience springs from the creative mind. Our thoughts about life create the outer effect we experience.

Not one thing exists that did not first exist as an idea in the imagination of someone. In out-of-body experiences we see that we exist outside of our physical body and can experience ourselves closer to the truth of who we are. We are pure consciousness, a composite of thought and feeling that is uniquely, individually, our self.

As we grow in awareness of the way in which we are creating our life's experience, we then can become conscious in the creative dream of objective reality. We can begin to integrate a higher aspect of our consciousness into our ego personality. We can then break down the artificial barriers separating the full range of our consciousness and begin to exert a conscious effect on our daily reality. When we can allow this to occur, we have begun to awaken to the reality of God within us, and to transcend our biological nature.

I present this to you as a picture of hope, for in this we can see our outward experiences are formed from our inner thoughts and feelings. It is we who are 100% responsible for our life. When we embrace this, we can begin to recreate it according to our wishes. Mind over matter is the reality. Matter is energy directed by thought, manifesting as matter. It is not a force of its own.

We must come to the recognition that with all illness, and particularly with AIDS, where our physical sciences offer no outward physical cure, we can look inwardly to the realms of thought and emotion and find the cause in the consciousness from which the disease springs. We can change the attitudes that do not serve us. When the limited thought in consciousness is removed, then the outer reality of disease must fall away into the nothingness from which it was made.

When there is a belief in an unlimited reality, out of this flows joy and peace. If every obstacle or condition must yield to the individual, then the doubt and fear manifesting as stress can not occur.

This belief in our unlimited potential, in a Christ-self, is the building block on which the individual must build his identity. It is the truth of his being. To accept less for ourself leads to the creation of negative emotions which suppress the barometer of joy, the immune system. When there is belief in limitlessness, there is hope. Where there is limitation, there is fear.

In Western society we have fallen victim to our sciences and our intellect. These systems deal only with the outer effect of our lives. The outer effect is not concrete reality. It is the projection of our belief systems onto reality. The physical surface of our life is the outgrowth of the internal reality from which it is created. The physical facts can be changed by changing the mental processes that cause the outer effect. We are not prisoners of the circumstances of our lives. We are their creator. But to claim our birthright we must first accept a new vision of ourselves.

The lowly caterpillar, with time, emerges from the cocoon a beautiful butterfly, transcending his earthbound self. The acorn has within it the mighty oak, which in time comes forth into expression. It cannot help but become the oak tree anymore than the caterpillar can prevent its wings from forming.

Within man is the potential of magnificence, the Christ awareness within - his true self. But God has given man free will. He must first accept the vision in order to become it. He is the only animal on the planet using but a small portion of his total brain. Why is it there? How is it activated? It is the mind without limit lying dormant, waiting for the acceptance that leads to its activation.

A greater thinking can be realized in the mind of man and a greater energy activated in the physical body. It can restore the immune system to a state of perfection no germ or virus can breach. Our ability to transcend our perceived limitations, as an aircraft speeding down a runway transcends the law of gravity, lies in our minds. As the law of lift takes over, it soars into flight. To claim our birthright we must first accept it as a possibility. Keeping in mind the knowledge of our true nature, we can then begin to take small steps towards it. Then the tailwinds of the universe will nudge us from behind toward the ultimate expression in our life. Not later, in some static heaven in the sky, but here and now in this life.

When man thinks of himself in strictly biological terms he has disconnected himself from his spiritual nature. This Nature is the source of his physical expression. It is then he finds himself a prisoner of the physical plane, a closed energy system which by definition must deteriorate and die. He has shut himself off from his connection to a universal and infinite energy supply which is by right his on which to draw. By an act of free will, a belief in his own mortality, he has chosen death.

If a deep sea diver where to become confused by what he saw as he peered through his mask onto the undersea world below, and were to release his connection to his air supply above, he would at some point run out of air and begin to drown. No amount of dissecting the fish and coral would give him a clue to the cause of his despair. He would have forgotten who he is and the source of his life giving oxygen. Only by reconnecting to his supply could he be saved.

This is the predicament of modern man. He has become disconnected from his spiritual life force. No amount of scientific examination of the world around him will give him the answer to his plight. The seemingly real world he dissects is but the physical effect of the projection of his own consciousness. He will not find the cause of his dis-ease outside himself. The true cause lies within his own consciousness and his rejection of his spiritual source. He must expand his awareness of himself to include his spiritual nature, a wholistic view of himself. Until man accepts his source he remains trapped in the physical dream, asleep to the miraculous potential that he is.

MIND – THE BUILDER

Our universe is one of energy expressing itself as matter. This matter is constantly pulsating, each physical object possessing a different vibrational frequency. A rock vibrates at a low frequency. Living matter vibrates at a higher frequency. These frequencies become increasingly high for electricity, light, and thought, which is the highest frequency of all.

Our thoughts are the tools by which we create our personal reality. Our thoughts do not end in our minds, but continue outward into other realities from which the physical world is created. By their electromagnetic frequencies, they magnetize to us the circumstances that mirror to us our thoughts.

Our experiences in life are formed by our beliefs about it. These beliefs are not facts about reality, but thoughts we have accepted to be true about it.

Our beliefs about reality create our expectations of our experience. Through our expectations we attract the events confirming our beliefs. We always experience our beliefs as the truth of our experience. Our beliefs are always confirmed by our experience. If we are to express ourselves as the power in our own lives, we must wake up and realize our beliefs form our experience.

Our beliefs create the expectations from which we act. We enter into the events of our lives with these expectations and we act, or react, in accordance with the beliefs from which they spring. The response we elicit from any circumstance will always mirror back to us our expectations about it.

Through thought we make choices which build the reality we experience; the circumstances of our life and health. It is through conscious awareness of these choices that we begin to awaken to our role as co-creators of our reality and of the universe.

Most of us have remained unconscious of our role as the creators of our own reality. We have allowed ourselves to be victimized by untamed minds running wild with thoughts of all kinds. As long as we are unconscious of their creative power and allow our thoughts to run unchecked, we will remain forever the victim of circumstances seemingly beyond our control. Until we begin to examine the contents of our own mind, we will continue asleep in the incarnational cycle of earth life.

In a lucid dream we become aware that the horrible nightmare we are experiencing is our own creation. We can awaken and find in reality we are in the safety of our own bed. So too can we awaken from the unconscious creation of our physical lives. We can discover we are safe indeed, and are the creators of our own reality.

Our experiences, whether in the dream state or what we call "real life", are creations of our minds. When we awaken to the truth of our unlimited reality, we can become the masters of our lives. The nightmare of AIDS is a creation of our unconscious use of thought. We can awaken from this as surely as the sleeping man awakens from his dream. We must awaken if we are to restore ourselves to health and happiness.

We carry on a constant dialogue in our head. At all times we are conversing with ourselves about whatever we are involved in at the time. We constantly reassess situations in the light of our beliefs about reality, and the constant dialogue in our minds reflect these beliefs. It is this constant chattering in our minds that reflects our belief systems and it is this internal mental dialogue that constantly affirms these beliefs. It is the tool by which we build our future experience moment by moment.

To become conscious creators of our reality we must become aware of this dialogue. Until we become conscious of what we are telling ourselves in each moment, we are at the mercy of our untamed mind. When we become consciously aware of the inner dialogue in our mind, we can begin to examine the beliefs by which we are building our future experience. We can then find the beliefs which serve to separate us from our true limitless ability to create for ourselves anything we desire. We can then gently replace them with new beliefs that will serve us in a better way. Through awareness of the inner dialogue we carry on with ourselves in our mind, we can begin to become the masters of our thoughts and thus the conscious creators of our lives.

As we begin to tune into our inner dialogue we will become aware of many different voices that speak to us at different times. Sometimes the voice of optimism can be heard. At other times we will hear the voice of doubt, or of guilt, or anger. Basically these voices can be placed into one of two categories. It is either the voice of love, which speaks in an affirmation of possibility, or the voice of fear, that speaks to us of limitation.

The voice of fear speaks to us out of our acceptance of limitation and will always reflect to us the limiting beliefs we hold about ourselves and about reality. It is the voice that denies we are the limitless creators of our own reality. It is the voice that says NO to our dreams and sows the seeds of doubt in us concerning our ability to create what we desire.

Fear always speaks of what might happen. It tries to convince us that we are at the mercy of forces beyond our control. It seeks to give our power away to situations outside ourself, to make us a victim of outer circumstances. It always speaks from the limiting beliefs we hold in consciousness and one by one closes the doors to a limitless life.

When we listen to the voice of fear, we begin to close ourselves off from the choices that are always before us. One by one, fear welds the bars onto the cage of limitation which it seeks to put us into. It is the voice that speaks to us of our belief in limitation. In truth, it has no more power over us than the energy we put into it.

If we are to quiet the voice of fear, we must examine the beliefs we hold in consciousness from which it draws its power. Do we believe we are the creators of our reality, or do we give away our power to outside circumstance? Do we accept abundance as the reality of life, or do we defer to scarcity? Is the AIDS virus all powerful and always fatal? Or is it we who are the co-creators of the universe and have the divine right to glowing health? It is beliefs such as these we must examine if we are to overcome the voice of fear.

To whatever degree we accept beliefs that limit our power, to that degree the voice of fear paralyzes us, preventing us from creating the life we desire. This fear and belief attract to us the very circumstances we dread so much and sets up reactions in our physical body that lower our immunity and lay us open to disease and death. The voice of fear is the voice of death.

The other voice that speaks to us from our inner dialogue is the voice of limitless love. It is the voice that speaks to us of possibility. Possibility creates feelings of joy. Whenever we have acted on a hunch and had that hunch come through, it was this voice which spoke to us. Or when we aimed for a goal and knew in our heart we could achieve it, it was this voice which told us it was so.

The voice that says YES to our deepest desires, that leaves us with joy in our heart, is the voice of limitless love. This voice speaks to us from the deepest truth of who we are. It is the voice speaking to us of our true relationship with the power that created the universe in which we have our very being. It will always seek to bring us into a greater realization of this relationship. It is the only voice whose power is rooted in reality. It is the voice of truth. It is not the voice that is heard first, however. It speaks in a whisper, and can only be heard through quiet listening.

Fear has no real power over us. It only has the power we give it through our belief in it. It only has the power of the limiting thoughts we have accepted for ourselves. As soon as we reject the beliefs in limitation, we begin to rob fear of its voice. When fear no longer has a voice from which to speak, we can bask in the reality of our deepest truth; the truth of our selves as a limitless beings of joy. We can then begin to hear the still small voice.

The Christ within, the realization of God in the form of a man, is the identity we awaken within ourselves when we begin to reject the identity of the altered ego - the voice distorted by limiting beliefs. As we examine the limitations we have accepted for ourselves and chose to hold or reject them, then we allow the universal flow toward fulfillment to manifest through us. It flows into our outer reality and we surrender into our metamorphosis. As the old identity falls away, we give birth to our inner truth which is the Christ-self within. We become fully awakened to our role as co-creator in the physical plane.

For the person faced with any fatal diagnosis and even more so with AIDS, which has so much of a stigma attached to it, the inner voice of fear is particularly strong. The acceptance of the medical community's beliefs about this disease, and all disease for that matter, has given fear a powerful voice. We are constantly bombarded by messages from a media which delights in the sensationalism of fear of this condition. We have accepted a view of disease based solely on the outer effect of the activity of germs and viruses. We have looked at the fate of others who have accepted this diagnosis and now fear it is our destiny to also die in like manner. We read the dire medical predictions the media sets forth and we adopt that fear as our own. But we have failed to see past the outer effect to the inner cause, which always lies within the consciousness of the "victim". The AIDS virus is only the physical mechanism by which the mental cause brings about its effect in biological reality.

If we were to attend a movie in which a murder was committed and then tried to change the action by rushing up to the screen, our effect at most would be to distort the picture. The murder would, however, continue. No amount of manipulation of the screen would cause the movie to unfold in a different manner. To change the story we would need to change the film in the projector. The picture is but a projection unto an empty screen.

The same is true of our lives. We experience the projection

of our belief systems onto the screen of our lives. It is the tape in our minds that must be changed if we are to ever truly affect real change in our lives. We must look at what we are projecting from our consciousness.

The challenge for the person with AIDS is to awaken and see through this illusion of illness. He can then begin to sift through the beliefs he has accepted about the process of disease and AIDS in particular. He can find the beliefs which do not serve his recovery. In doing this, he can stop his progress dictated by the medical blueprint for death and begin to restore himself to wholeness.

If we were to stand with our nose pressed up against a painting in the impressionistic style, what we would see would be many disconnected dots. They would seem to have no meaning or relationship to each other or a larger picture. However, as we begin to stand back from the canvas and observe from a broader prospective, we would begin to see a different picture emerge. We would perceive the slashes of color in relationship to each other and the picture as a whole. This is what we can do with our lives and the seemingly separate events in it. We can step back and view them from a different perspective. Then we will begin to see relationships and patterns in a way that relates to the larger canvas of our life. For healing we must enlarge our perception of reality and of ourselves.

The fear that tells us there is no hope speaks from the power of limiting beliefs. It only has the power we choose to give it. When we know the truth about reality and ourselves, we can begin to see past the outer illusions of life. We can look within our mind and see the seeds we have planted, that have sprouted into the outer effects of our life. And we can know for sure that we are the creators of our reality and have the power to recreate it in any way we desire. Our awareness of our inner dialogue will show us the beliefs from which we have created our circumstance. We can then root out those that have limited us in any way.

We must begin to listen to the thoughts constantly passing through our mind. As we become aware of the voice of fear that speaks to us of limitation, we can recognize it and use it as a flag for underlying beliefs giving it power. We can then, through our awareness of the belief, gently remind ourself of our desired belief in limitlessness. By consistent awareness of our inner dialogues we can begin to re-program our consciousness with new beliefs of our choosing. As these beliefs take root in our consciousness, we begin to act out of them. They will ripple outward from us to change the reality of our lives.

We live in a benevolent universe. It has a propensity to push us in the direction of fulfillment and health. It is this propensity for good that causes a wild flower to push its way through the asphalt of a road. In human consciousness it is our acceptance of limitations that is the asphalt covering the bloom of health and abundance. We can begin to move past our limits through awareness of our inner dialogue.

EMOTION

Belief is translated into health or disease through the emotional body. Each belief held in consciousness produces a corresponding emotion that is, at its essence, electrical energy. This energy is felt in the body as emotion. These emotions in turn activate the physical body through the glands of the endocrine system. These glands are the physical mechanism by which spirit meets matter, by which belief, through emotion, creates physical health or disease in the body.

The hormonal secretions of the endocrine system have direct impact upon the major organs with which they are associated. The immune system, whose function is controlled by these secretions, is either stimulated or suppressed. The immune system is the measure of joy in the body. It is this system that is attacked and destroyed by AIDS.

The glands of the endocrine system correspond to the seven chakras in the body. These chakras, or energy centers in the body, are motivational centers and are triggered into activity by the various emotional states in man. When out of balance, the four lower chakras relate to the negative emotions - fear, anger, guilt, envy, and unforgiveness. Whatever emotional attitude is being expressed, the corresponding center, with its glands and organs, is affected.

By mastering these emotional states, exercising the choice of love over fear, the lower four centers are brought into balance and the upper three chakras of the body are activated. These upper chakras relate to the activation of the dormant portions of the brain and the awakening of man as a conscious creator of his reality, able to manifest his desires. The activation of the unused portions of the brain lead to total limitlessness. By mastering fear and its accompanying emotions, through the expression of love, man begins to transcend his biological cocoon and to realize in himself his divine unlimited nature.

Until man has achieved mastery over the lower four centers which trap him in limited human experience, these upper three chakras can not be safely activated. These lower four energy centers must be balanced if man is to restore health to the body. These four centers, when activated by fear and its related emotions, produce the poisonous glandular secretions inhibiting immune response. This allows disease conditions to develop.

Without mastery of negativity, man remains a victim of viruses and germs, a frail biological creature attacked from without and within by a hostile environment over which he seemingly has no control. Negativity robs man of his birthright as a limitless being of health and abundance. These negative emotions are produced by limiting beliefs.

Emotions, whether negative or positive, must be allowed expression. Through expression we maintain the flow of life-force through our physical bodies. When we lack self-love and hold beliefs limiting our ability to express our feelings, this lack of expression holds the electrical current of the emotion within the body. This current then continuously acts upon the corresponding energy center in the body. These centers, through their physical counterparts, the glands of the endocrine system, produce hormonal secretions which can be either beneficial or poisonous. The secretions act directly upon the organs associated with each center. The expression, "To vent your spleen," literally draws on ancient knowledge of the interaction of the emotional and physical bodies. Similarly, "To eat ones heart out," shows the same.

The first step in healing is to allow the emotional body expression. To fail to do so is to literally rob the body of vitality and make it fertile ground for the actions of germs and viruses.

The electrical currents of emotions act not only upon the energy centers of the physical body through which disease processes are initiated. They are also the mechanism by which belief creates the experienced reality. Emotional feeling is expressed as electrical current outwardly through the auric field, which is the energy field surrounding the physical body. These electrical values then act as a magnetic field to draw toward the individual, experiences of like emotional values. In other words, it attracts experiences that will reflect back what one feels to be true. In this two-fold manner, emotion, flowing out of belief, is the mechanism by which thought is translated into health in the body as its first reflection. It then attracts the body of life experience.

When the emotions are not allowed expression then the ability to perceive clearly what is happening in the present moment is clouded. Our perceptions become distorted by the feelings we hold around a circumstance. As we begin to allow expression of our feelings, we gain clarity of mind and limit their impact on the body. With this clarity, we can search for the judgments and beliefs we hold which cause the unwanted emotional response. We can choose to let go of the beliefs that do not serve us. The judgments we hold are the cause of all emotional reaction. They in turn attract our experiences. Through the release of judgment we begin to heal the emotional body and release the physical experience.

The acorn does not insist it is only a seed and refuse to burst forth into its full potential as a mighty oak. If it held to a strict definition of itself as a seed and denied itself expansion, it would rot and die on the ground, never achieving its potential as a tree. Instead, it lets nature define it. It blooms into a magnificent oak, becoming the potential that always was within. The same is true with man. When he claims he is only human and refuses to accept the limitless potential of the Christ-self within, he has blocked the expression of his true nature. He remains forever just a man, with all of the weakness of the flesh.

Man has free will and he can choose freedom for himself.

He cannot be forced into acceptance against his will. Consciousness constantly nudges him toward his potential but it is a choice each person must make for themselves in the end. AIDS is an opportunity to make this choice, and a most dramatic one. It is a chance to examine our self perceptions, becoming more than we have allowed ourselves to be. Or we can choose to remain with our limited definitions of self and suffer the consequences.

Growth, change, and expression are constants in life. AIDS can be a mechanism by which to achieve all three. To see the opportunity is a choice we must make for ourselves, however. We must let go of our limiting definitions of who we are and reach for limitless life.

When man rejects the belief in his limitless self and accepts beliefs about himself and life that limit him in any way, he experiences fear. It does not matter whether the beliefs are religious, scientific, or societal in nature. Fear is produced by any perception of self that says it is not in control, a belief things have a cause outside of self.

The belief that we are acted upon by things beyond our control produces fear. Anger is a belief that something has been done to us by another. Envy springs from a belief in lack. Guilt is produced when we judge ourselves for our perceived failures. All of these emotions are a result of our ignorance of the truth. They are all produced by false assumptions about ourselves and reality.

All perceptions based on these false assumptions are distorted. When we base our life's choices on false information about ourself and reality, then the resulting experience is a distortion of reality. The degree to which we acquiese to power outside of ourselves is the degree to which we experience less than our birthright of health and abundance.

If we are to master the emotions manifesting through the body as disease, we must first correct our false assumptions about who we are. We must accept that we are the creator of our reality without limitation, and turn to this belief when a question of action arises. We must set the unlimited potential of Christ within as the ideal.

There is nothing to fear. We live as limitless beings in a universe of good intent, ever striving to bring us into that full realization. But only we can let go of the faulty definitions that we have accepted of our self, that block our full expression.

The emotion of fear, and all of its resulting negative effects, is created out of the false assumptions on which mankind has built his history and civilization. Our society today is based upon the assumption that man is a biological creature only. We believe we must wrestle our needs from a hostile environment. Our myths and religions, which speak of our greater identity, have been pushed aside as nothing but primitive superstitions. The rational intellectual mind has been chosen over man's intuitive nature, as if feeling were somehow less real than facts.

Man's myths and religions are not superstitions, but attempts to express a long forgotten truth about who he really is. He is a limitless entity expressing in a physical body, with an existence anchored in realities beyond the physical dimensions of time and space. He is not the product of an accidental mixing of the primeval soup, resulting in this chance existence we call life. He is the creator of his own reality, a victim of nothing but ignorance of his true power. He is a God accepting limitation, hypnotized by that acceptance into experiencing it as reality.

The lack and disease mankind faces are but illusions supported by the energy he channels into them, by his acceptance of them as real. If he is to conquer the fear creating these experiences then he must take a leap of faith and accept the possibility of being 100% responsible for his experience. He must at the very least be willing to accept he can become the limitless creator of his own reality. Without this acceptance, his reaction to his perceived reality will continue to be based on false assumptions about himself. His reactions and experience will continue to be distorted.

When man begins to examine his beliefs and circumstance in light of a new understanding of his identity, then he can begin to let go of the fear and anger that produce disease in his body and chaos in the body of his life. When he recognizes the limitless possibilities lying dormant in each moment of any situation he faces, then the stress that produces anxiety, fear, and anger can begin to ebb.

All negativity is produced by a belief in limitation. The acceptance of this limitation, expressing as negative emotion, reacts in the physical body through the glands of the endocrine system. These glands are then triggered to secrete the hormones which act to suppress or over activate immune response. When immune response is exhausted by this continual activation or suppression, then the organs of the body begin to deteriorate and the entire system is exposed to the action of germs and virus. The result is disease and deterioration of the physical body.

False belief lies at the root of the illusionary realities of illness and lack. Those beliefs in limitation produce the emotions of negativity that act on the body through the endocrine system to produce disease. We accept arbitrary judgments of good and bad, success and failure, instead of seeing all experience as leading to growth. By our judgment we accept only a narrow range of experience as acceptable, cutting ourself off from our truest desires by faulty rationalizations. We let guilt and fear of failure wrench our birthright away from us.

The power disease has over us is an illusion born of our beliefs in limitation. We then do battle with the illusion, boxing with a shadow, all the while ignoring the greater cause. For every symptom suppressed, larger ones are created until with AIDS, we can go no further with the game. We must face at last the cause in consciousness.

Disease is a message from consciousness, spoken by the body. It needs to be faced with love, not suppressed out of fear. When we love ourselves totally because we know who we are, we love and accept our body's message. We then embrace its lesson.

Our bodies do not speak to us in a foreign tongue, but through the energetic language of the chakra system. This is ancient knowledge. It sounds foreign to us only because we have moved so far away from a true understanding of our reality and ourselves. We need to explore who we really are. We will find a sleeping God in human form.

Discovering the God within produces a feeling called joy. Joy, and its fellow emotions of love and laughter, react on the endocrine system in a different way than fear. They react to produce the life giving hormonal secretions that promote healthy organs and immune response. Norman Cousins found this truth and laughed his way to health from his deathbed of cancer. By letting go of our limited beliefs and assumptions about life and letting our self evolve beyond the limited imaginings of the human mind, we too can laugh at AIDS and walk away from the illusion of certain death.

The man who dares to dream his own dream and to know he is the limitless creator that brings the dream into reality for himself, will become an aspect of the God he seeks. He who allows no other person or belief to thwart his self expression, will become a unique expression of the God within him. By the release of judgment and the expression of the self's truest desires, genius is ours to own.

THE LAW OF KARMA

There is a universal law which is fundamental to all existence. Whether one understands this underlying principle in terms of belief creating reality, experience as a projection of consciousness, or a law of physics, it is all the same. This law is the law of karma. Jesus described it so well 2000 years ago when he said, "Whatsoever a man shall sow, that shall he reap." He knew conclusively that the universe in which we live is neither accidental nor random. We are victims of nothing save the harvest of our own planting. An understanding of this law is imperative to the attaining of a stance in life that will allow us to move into an ever greater expression of abundance and health.

We are the generators of our own experience. We are not passive spectators in the drama of our own lives, either in the form or the essence it takes. The collection of beliefs and attitudes composing the contents of our own consciousness are mirrored back to us in the events of our life. No circumstance we are presented with comes to us except it be a reflection of a thought or action that we ourselves have initiated. By attraction we pull to us the circumstances which will act as lessons to best teach us about ourselves. Karmic law is how we create the perfect situations to advance us in our spiritual growth.

When we resist the lessons with which we present ourselves, we have assumed an inverted stance toward life. To react against a situation is to set in motion yet another event of like value, until the decision is reached to face the circumstance and embrace the lesson it offers. Through loving acceptance the cycle of karma is broken.

There is a law of physics which states, "for every action there is an equal and opposite reaction." This physical law is a reflection of the universal law of karma. It can be seen in operation in both the physical and mental realms.

When I was a child, there was a fierce dog in my neighborhood, of which I was deathly afraid. Each time I would come anywhere near the dog I would recoil in fear. Each time the dog would try to attack me. I noticed, however, that some people could approach the dog and get a friendly response. In my mind it was perhaps their familiarity to the dog that made this possible. Finally, someone took the time to explain to me that if I would approach the dog in a non-defensive manner, without reacting in fear, then the dog's response would be different. Sure enough, when I approached the dog without fear, he responded in a friendly manner. This was a lesson I have seen in operation in all aspects of my own life.

On a daily basis we experience this type of immediate karmic response in our dealings with one another. Each time we come face-to-face with another person we have an opportunity to observe this law in action. If we approach each other with openness, not bringing into the present situation any judgments based on past experience, then the response to us is that same openness. If we choose not to forgive the past, and bring an attitude based on previous experience into the present situation, then we recreate the past experience over again in the present. In either case, the response we attract is dependent on how we choose to approach the situation.

When we hold old images of one another, we continue to project them onto each other even though they no longer fit the present situation. By Karmic law that projection will be mirrored back to us by our experiences with one another.

Fear invites attack. To act in fear toward something is indicative of a belief in a lack of safety. This belief is always reflected back to us as an attack on our person. A defensive attitude shows a belief there is a need to be protected from something. It draws attack to us.

Our military build-up testifies to our belief as a nation in the lack of safety this world affords. In truth, the armaments we create for our own protection have created the enemy from which we must now protect ourself. The outer surface of our life as individuals and societies always mirrors back to us our beliefs. We have forgotten the enemy has been created by our own fear and defensiveness, not the other way around. The threat we see around the globe to our own safety is a mirror of our own fear.

The thinking of the world is an inversion of the truth. This is the thinking that has given us the arms race as a means of securing peace. It has given us "peacekeeping missiles" and atomic overkill. This thought pattern is insane.

We have become reactive rather than creative in our stance toward life. We have forgotten who we are and the power of our own minds in creating the very realities we then react to. We are battling effects, the cause of which lies in our own thought processes.

Weapons are created to be used. They never contribute to peace. They create the resistance which then must be defended against. "Those who live by the sword will die by the sword" is a restatement of karmic law. Peace cannot be secured by military might. Only war is created by military might.

Peace is created by loving acceptance for all life. It is not created by forcing others to live according to a set of rules not to their liking. When we "love our enemies," then we have no enemies. When love is extended, then by the law of karma only love is returned. It is the only power that can possibly establish peace.

A view of American foreign policy would give an excellent illustration of this type of inverted thinking. In country after country, dictatorial governments backed by U.S. support have been toppled or threatened by insurgencies of a religious or political nature. As a national policy we pour more and more arms and money into propping up these regimes.

These are regimes that almost always enforce the kind of

repression we as a nation would not possibly condone for ourselves. Yet we continue to degrade our own principles of freedom by our actions in other lands because of our insane inverted logic.

But one-by-one these unpopular leaders have been over-thrown and incredible outbursts of anti-American feelings have followed. We then order larger outlays of money and armaments to fight the threat, but it ominously continues to grow. We are caught up in a karmic cycle of our own making.

An underlying assumption to a policy such as this is that it is necessary to suppress the rights of others in order to secure our own interests. We perceive our own interest as different from others. We use elaborate excuses to condone that the end justifies the means in the case of our own self interest. We help establish regimes that suppress the masses of their own people, but which will support policies we deem in our best interest. Our support of oppression ferments the dissatisfaction which ultimately grows into a rebellious insurgency against us. We then pour even more resources into defending against that threat.

The understanding needed here is that the threat is self-created. It is never in our own interest to suppress another's rights. It is suppression that creates the resistance. It is only in our interest to allow for all men that which we desire for ourselves.

If all the money spent to prop up these dictators were used to educate people so they could grow to be self-sufficient, then there would be no fertile soil in which a communist insurgency could ferment. The pursuit of a positive focus such as this would create loving feelings toward our real interests. Instead, to the oppressed citizens of these countries, communist help becomes the means of salvation from the lack of freedom we have forced upon them. We have made ourselves the enemy and pushed away those we need as allies into the opposing camp. All of this is a result of karmic law.

You serve your own interest by serving the interest of others, not by opposing it. You must extend to others what you would have for yourself. What you would hoard will be taken from you.

The old formulas of strength through might will increasingly fail as we approach the new millennium. We must heal the erroneous perceptions of our minds. Loving support must replace selfish exploitation or we as a nation will soon be forced to face the harvest of our sowing.

At the end of WW II, in one of the most magnanimous gestures in the history of the world, the United States helped rebuild the war ravaged countries of Western Europe, including Germany and Japan, against whom we had fought. The result of this extension of support, called the Marshall Plan, was to usher in a post-war era of prosperity the likes of which had never been seen before. This act of cooperation opened and established markets for U.S. goods that would not have otherwise existed. To this day they are essential to the healthy functioning of our own economy. With this selfless act of giving we created for ourselves the prosperity we now enjoy.

We chose not to react with hostility against our wartime enemies, but to forgive and to create for ourselves, through the service of others, a better future for all. This is the thinking which is life-enhancing. This is what we have lost as a nation and as individuals, and it is threatening to take all we value away from us.

We are the only ones who can change the doomsday scenarios now approaching because we are the ones who have created them. When we act from the root assumptions of lack of safety and scarcity, we create that reflection in the body of our lives.

Edgar Cayce described karma as the meeting of self. As creators of reality that is just what we are experiencing in our daily lives. Karma is the law and must be met. To give is to receive, being polarities of the same action. To defend is to create attack. Karma is not imposed on us from the outside against our will. If is self-generated by the projection of our own attitudes.

There is but one way in which karma can be met and transmuted. That is through loving acceptance of the lessons it brings. To resist or deny the lessons is but to create another of increasing intensity until at some point we choose to learn the lessons it would teach. All of the events of our life are lessons born out of the attitudes we hold in consciousness. The purpose of these lessons is not to punish us, but to move our thinking into closer alignment with truth.

We must choose to face our karma with loving acceptance for the lesson we have created. Then we have created a way in which the experience can be released so as to become a stepping stone in our own evolution. We are never presented with a lesson which does not have inherent within it a way to learn from the situation and then release it and move beyond.

The one thing we can be sure of is that each situation in life contains a gift within it. We do not experience it when we choose to resist or deny the lesson. This only locks us into a reactive stance which ties us to the wheel of karma. Then we continually recreate the same pattern in our life over and over again.

To face every circumstance we are presented with loving acceptance for the lesson it would teach, knowing we have created the perfect opportunity for our own growth, is to break free of the karmic cycle and to take the creative role in our own experience. Loving acceptance of life and of each other is the path to transcending the pain of this world.

As we meet karma with love, learning the lessons it brings, we grow to a point in consciousness where it is no longer necessary for us to create painful lessons from which to learn. Now, because we have projected nothing but loving acceptance in each circumstance we have faced, by karmic law nothing but love will begin to return to us. The mirror of life can only reflect the consciousness we project onto it. It would be impossible to meet with anything but love. It is now we can begin the process of growth through joy and fulfillment.

To transcend the law of karma is to bring your life experience under the law of grace. To live from the God within, which is that place of loving acceptance within each and everyone of us, is to live in abundance and health amid a world that believes in sickness and lack. To give only loving acceptance to all things is to experience life from the God-awareness of your own consciousness. It is to see only love everywhere and in all things.

This awareness allows us to have our needs met by the attractive force we have become. "All things work together for good to them that love God" is the realization that you already have everything you need or it is on its way. This is the understanding that allows one to release the belief in stress and struggle. To live from the God within is to have only love reflected back in our experience and that is peace and health and joy.

The opportunity for the release from karma exists in each moment through the person or circumstance before us. To extend love in each moment is to live from the awareness of our limitless nature. This is the path to freedom. To extend love to others is the only way to receive more for oneself. Love is never decreased by extending, it is only increased. Love is lost by withholding it because then there is none. Love is felt only in the sharing. To understand this is the secret of inner peace.

DISEASE

In the traditional medical approach to health and the body, we find a heavy concentration on germs as the cause of disease. Someone has a cold and sneezes, spewing germs in the air. The next unsuspecting fellow passing by unwittingly takes the germ into his body and is attacked, quickly coming down with a cold. This would seem hard to deny and yet, what of those who take in the germ and remain disease free?

Over a million men and women are exposed to the AIDS virus and yet we see only a percentage of those exposed going on to develop full-blown AIDS. Others remain incubating for a time and then succumb, while others never exhibit any symptoms at all. What we need to explore here is not the disease process, but why one person remains well while the other succumbs.

We need to expand our understanding of the role germs and viruses play in the biological process of life. No life would exist without their presence. They have a benevolent role to play.

A virus is very similar to a crystal in nature. It responds according to the energy environment in which it finds itself. It is triggered into a level of activity that is disease producing by the environment. Exposure to the virus is not the real issue with AIDS. Rather the question one so infected might ask himself is "Why does this virus respond so destructively to the environment in my body?"

We need to deal with the cause of our internal environment. It is the anger, frustration, and resentment created by thought systems held in consciousness we must address. When we deal with these issues, an environment is created within the body in which the virus can be restored to a more appropriate level of activity.

When a person has immunity from a disease, it is mental immunity that he first has. He has resisted the thoughts which give rise to the attitudes and emotions from which disease is born. When there is an epidemic such as the AIDS crisis we now face, it is first an epidemic of belief. One person falls victim and the next does not. It is the consciousness of the individual that provides the immunity. The germ is the physical vehicle by which consciousness creates the condition.

In the light of the truth of man as creator of his reality through the content of his conscious mind, let us look at the way in which the process of disease emerges in man. Unlimited man exists in abundance and health. The Christ-self lies as his potential within. It is man at the point of God, all knowingness, man with a fully activated brain. He experiences no fear for he is totally aware he is the creator of his life experience. He is awake in the reincarnational dream of physical existence. How did this unlimited man become the limited self he is today? Through judgment of his experiences.

In the allegory in the book of Genesis, man ate of the fruit of the tree of knowledge of good and evil and was cast out of the garden into a life of limitation. It was judgment that cut man off from his true nature. Man has struggled toward the release of judgment since his existence here began.

Out of judgment grew the emotions known as fear and guilt, the most paralyzing and useless emotions of all. From these came all other emotions of anger, unforgiveness, envy, and resentment. By the laws of consciousness these emotions create for man the very situations he fears. Man's fear materializes itself so he can face it and go through the nothingness that it is. He can then begin to learn once again of his limitlessness.

Disease is one of the mechanisms by which conscious brings error in thought to light, in order for it to be examined. When man does not face his fears, they are reflected in the body as stress. Stress is what replaces the joy that is his birthright.

The physical body is man's most immediate creation and it is the first reflection of the mind. His beliefs create the emotional contents of his life. His limited beliefs create the negative emotions he feels. They are energy blockages in the path of the life-force coursing through him. Through the imbalances this creates in the chakra system of the body, the corresponding organs and glands are impacted and the free flow of energy through them is reduced. These areas of reduced energy-flow then become the areas in which germs and viruses, which are always present, can become triggered into destructive activity.

With our medical sciences we have learned to suppress symptoms to a limited degree. If the root cause in consciousness is not removed however, disease will manifest again in other ways. When we refuse to deal with the root causes and deal only with the outward symptoms, which are the outgrowth of the mental cause, consciousness will create ever larger roadblocks. In that respect our medical sciences actually create ever larger disease conditions by suppressing symptoms. The afflicted then delays the examination of his consciousness, in which the symptoms have their source. This creates the necessity for another symptom of greater magnitude.

When we truly give ourselves love and acceptance, then our view of illness can change. We can begin to accept the messages our physical body is giving us. Symptoms are how the body speaks to us. When we ignore its message, we are not loving our bodies fully. When we accept our illness for the lesson it is teaching, this will bring the change in consciousness which will allow the experience to be released. Our experiences are the three dimensional effects of our consciousness. When we deal with the cause, the effect must flow from our experience.

An examination of the progression of venereal disease as it relates to the gay community will show a progression from minor annoyances, such as crabs and gonorrhea, to syphilis, to amebiasis, to AIDS, each disease increasing in severity and difficulty to cure. It is but a trail of roadblocks consciousness has created in an effort to have the root causes examined.

As each symptom is suppressed, delaying examination of the real cause, then a new one is created in increasing intensity until it has culminated in AIDS, which demands that we stop and examine ourselves. To not do so is to die. Consciousness has manifested this disease in such a way that it cannot be suppressed with a pill. It forces us to deal with the true cause in order to find relief.

We have been afraid to look within at the cause for fear AIDS is a judgment on our sexuality. It is not. It does speak to our loveless use of the body, however. AIDS is offering us an opportunity to change. It is seeking to bring us into closer alignment with love. If we try to ignore its message with our medicines, would we really want to see the next degree to which consciousness will go in its demand to be examined? I think not.

Life is a flow. It is a movement by which spiritual inspiration, felt in the heart as feelings, gives us the surest course of action to take in the expression of our lives. This inspiration comes from our spiritual self, existing outside time and space and our physical body. It gives us the knowledge of our purpose and path to fulfillment.

It is the role of the ego personality, the self we know in this physical reality, to act upon the feelings of the heart. It serves to bring them into outward expression in our lives. This flow or movement, from the internal inspiration to the outward expression, is the essence of life itself.

In nature the flow is unimpeded. In man, the conscious mind, the ego personality, becomes the filter regulating the allowance of this flow. Through the altering of the ego, by the acceptance of beliefs that limit the expression of spiritual inspiration, the flow and movement that is life itself is slowly cut off. The resulting blockage, in pure energy terms, is what we have come to know as disease.

The ego mind in its altered state of limitation becomes the

blockage in the process of self-becoming, self-expression. The seed does not become the oak. The caterpillar never gets its wings. The embryo is aborted. Death and disease are the result.

Disease is a message from our physical bodies that something is wrong with our perceptions. To attack the symptom is not to give the body acceptance of its message. This is to give the body only conditional love and acceptance. It is not the way to create healing.

Healing is allowed when the symptoms are faced and the message accepted. It is then that the experience of disease can be released. When the cause in consciousness is resolved, the physical experience is dissolved.

We must look to the root cause of denial of true self, from which all disease springs. The soul is demanding love of self through illness. It will not be denied. Without love from itself, it will cease to sustain physical life.

To transcend disease, we must balance the emotions from which it originates; emotions of fear, anger, and unforgiveness. We must examine the beliefs from which illness springs, not suppress their outer effects. We must examine the limiting beliefs, both personal and medical, we have accepted for ourselves. We must begin to look beyond the symptoms and the sciences that have grown up around them, to the internal seeds in which they have their source.

The body is a marvelous creation. It has the ability to maintain itself in perfect working order at all times. It is indeed a wonderous marvel of complexity which no man-made machine can hope to rival. And yet we experience sickness and pain. We have come to see ourselves as frail victims of dangers lurking everywhere in germs and viruses. These viruses have a benevolent intent in the physical cooperation of life and yet, we have made them our enemies.

We have blocked the flow of health through our bodies by the dirty window of limiting belief our consciousness has become. We have not accepted our birthright of health and joy. We have blocked it at every turn. We must begin to root out the beliefs that block this flow and allow glowing health to manifest once again in our bodies and lives. We must say yes to our true identity so we can begin the most exciting journey of becoming ourselves. For this is life - the journey into awareness of who we truly are. We must accept who we are and begin to allow it. To refuse is to remain in sickness and lack.

By rejecting the limitations of the ego and saying yes to the deepest desires of our hearts, we can step by step begin to increase the flow of the life force through our physical bodies. We can transcend, through love, the actions of germs and viruses and manifest glowing health.

In the case of AIDS, where science has little to offer, we must open our minds to the greater possibilities that lie within. The healer within is the God within. When we connect to our inner source, the physical healing we seek will manifest. When we become our whole self, our bodies will reflect back to us our inner wholeness.

There will not be a magic pill to cure AIDS. Like cancer before it, the billions we have spent on medical research have not provided a cure. We have not been aware of their true cause. Both AIDS and cancer demand a wholistic approach to treatment, not just in terms of alternate physical therapies. They both demand spiritual awakening. These diseases have their true origin in the mind and spirit. It is there we must seek the cure.

MESSAGES OF AIDS

Each of us chooses to experience many lifetimes in physical reality. We incarnate into different cultures, languages, and mindsets. Through the contexts of these various experiences, we develop within ourselves the self love necessary to propel us into a full expression of our spiritual nature. Each life experience offers to us the maximum potential for achieving this goal.

We choose our sex and parents, our country, and our physical bodies. We also choose the circumstances that will allow us the greatest opportunity to learn in physical reality, our true identity of limitlessness. We then incarnate as babes into the dream of physical life, to journey from forgetfulness of our true selves into full self-realization.

One of the many expressions we choose is homosexual. It is but one path needed that the soul might come to know itself. It is a noble path made exceedingly difficult by the judgments our society, religions, and scientific communities have made against this choice.

Perhaps no other aspect of life has been so distorted and judged against as sexuality. To grow up homosexual in this society is to be bombarded from the earliest age with messages making self-esteem an impossibility. Our religious institutions declare it to be "an abomination against God." The secular segments of society engage in serious debate over the question of basic human rights for the homosexual, as if that debate were a serious question of moral judgment.

Yet clearly the scriptures upon which Christainity rest tells us, "Judge not that ye be not judged. "It is neither our responsibility, nor within our ability, to make these judgments for another. Rather, we are to extend love and support toward all, not excluding those we have judged undeserving. Our nation's constitution states that all men are created equal and yet not only homosexuals, but racial minorities and women have had to risk life and limb to wrestle even the slightest of basic rights from the establishment.

Homosexuality is a true expression of the soul. To deny it is to deny one's self. For many years, those in the gay community accepted the judgments placed upon them by others and therefore experienced those judgments accordingly. Acceptance of these judgments led in times past to overwhelming feelings of self-loathing and helped to create the stereotype of the lonely and pitiful homosexual. In the past many generations of homosexuals have lived this cruel lie. In the acceptance of these judgments placed on them by others, they judged themselves.

The acceptance of these judgments produces feelings of guilt which always seek to be punished. Many homosexuals have lived lives of misery and self-hate because of this. The alcoholism, promiscuity, and drug abuse seen in the gay community are all outer forms indicative of the severity of these inner psychic wounds.

To grow up in an environment which extends no love or support but instead offers only condemnation, makes the self-esteem necessary for a healthy functioning life nearly impossible. Without love, a healthy life is not possible. Even with all of their necessary physical needs met, babies abandoned by their parents in institutions do not live without being nurtured and supported and loved. If they do survive, they grow up to be twisted adults. Much of the destructive behavior seen in the homosexual community comes from a basic lack of self-love which has grown from the acceptance of these brutal judgments society has made against us.

The gay community does not exist in isolation however.

AIDS serves the purposes of both the homosexual and heterosexual communities. It allows those who are disenfranchised from the whole of society a way out of an unbearable situation. In dying they are able to make a statement to both the gay community and society at large of the price to be paid by all for a lack of loving acceptance. These deaths serve as a warning to each of us of the need to examine our attitudes toward our sexuality and one another.

AIDS is not a punishment from God for the alleged perversion of homosexuality as some fundamentalists have claimed. That judgment merely reflects their own issues of guilt and shame around sexuality. It is in truth their own self-judgment. This judgment and guilt are the fertile soil that will attract to them this experience. This judgment and lack of compassion continues to pull AIDS further into the mainstream experience. The fear now beginning to permeate the consciousness of the masses concerning AIDS is a creative force. This fear will draw to them the thing they have most judged against.

There is only one solution to this dilemma. If AIDS wipes out half the population of the entire earth, those who remain will have gotten the point. It is that we are one people on one planet. The only proper response to one another is loving allowance and acceptance. The hell of AIDS is not the wrath of God on a cursed people. It is the manifested creation of mankind's misaligned thinking.

In 1969 the blessed day of Stonewall liberation came and homosexuals began at last to stand up and speak the truth of who they were. This new self-acceptance brought joy into many lives. The gay community was finally able to express without fear of reprisal those aspects of itself that had been denied for so long. This was a great step forward. To deny one's self-expression is to live a lie. Lies have consequences.

For many people, however, there has been the over-identification with the label of homosexuality. Many limiting judgments have been attached to it by this generation. The normal expression of our sexuality has become a limiting "lifestyle" leading to the defining of homosexuality in strictly sexual terms. This is a lie in light of the true identity of the self as a limitless whole. To define oneself in terms of only one small aspect of the whole only is to accept limitation. To then use that limited identity to create a separation from the whole of self and the whole society of which one is a part, is to be psychically fragmented. The truth of one's wholeness will always seek to triumph over an image.

With AIDS, it is not necessarily the expression of the homosexual's soul that cries out for change. It is only our sexual expression seeking a greater expansion. It is the embracing of homosexuality as a limitation that needs to be changed in our minds. We must first reject the limited image we have accepted. Then we must accept the larger truth of ourselves. Only we can do that. By accepting wholeness we can allow it to express in our experience. By holding the ideal in mind, we can move forward into health.

We are not wrong in our sexual expression, yet we have embraced limited meanings about who we are. The attachment of limited definitions to homosexuality cause us to view ourselves as isolated from the whole of humanity and our greater self. This then limits our fullest expression. It is imperative we accept our whole identity as the truth of our being. We must stop defining ourselves by just one small aspect of this whole. We must allow homosexuality to become one adjective in many by which we express our whole truth. Our sexuality must be integrated as an aspect of our personality, and not be allowed to dominate it.

The separation from society we as homosexuals experience is a reflection of the segmentation within our own souls. In seeking to establish a sense of self-esteem in the midst of a society that rejects us totally, we have taken that rejection and inverted it in our minds into a sense of specialness. We have used a ghetto mentality to create a sense of superiority toward those who have oppressed us. The end result is still the same separation.

When there is separation there is isolation, and isolation invites attack. When there is limitation there is fear, and fear invites attack. Limitation and fear do not produce the joy of which our own bodies immune system is the measure. Some doctors will tell you it is normal for the T-cell count of a homosexual to be lower than that of the average heterosexual person. It is not normal. It is the reflection in the physical body of the loss of joy in the soul created by separation.

There exists as great an animosity in the gay community towards heterosexuals as exists the other way around. Both segments mirror back to each other the judgments they hold about each other. We are locked in a karmic embrace that must be broken. This will only come when each side begins to accept the other and to focus on our commonalties instead of our differences. The end product of the old sentiments is the AIDS epidemic we are now experiencing.

How far this will spread is a decision each of us will help to make. In the end, no amount of latex will protect us. HIV and all viruses are present in each and every person on this planet. They are necessary to the biological processes of life. They are activated to destructive power by the hatred in men's hearts.

We must begin to see AIDS as a cry for love by a minority segment of society. It is a plea to the greater whole in a desperate attempt for love and acceptance. Until we understand this, this plague will continue to grow. This is one gift of the disease called AIDS. When it has run its course we shall all be changed people, one people on one planet. The form this change finally takes is dependent upon how long it takes us to learn the lessons.

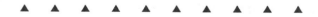

If we are to examine AIDS as it relates to the homosexual community in light of spiritual truth, then we must look at how and where the disease is manifesting. First of all, we find that it is transmitted through bodily fluids in intimate sexual activity and that exposure does not necessarily indicate whether a person will develop the disease or not. A small percentage will develop the full-blown syndrome resulting in a gradual wasting death while many will exhibit only mild symptoms (ARC) and others will show no signs of infection at all.

One of the contributing factors resulting in full blown infection is repeated exposure to the virus. Let us examine promiscuity as it relates to self-denial and the avoidance of intimacy. On the flip side of any problem always lies the answer. We must look deeper at this issue to find the clues we seek.

It is not the repetition of any act in itself that causes full blown infection. There is no judgment of any sexual act. Surely we have known those that have frequent partners and continue to be well, while others engaging in less sexual activity have died. It is the consciousness the person brings into the sexual act, that lies at the root of the problem.

For many promiscuity has become a lifestyle. It has its roots in the inability of the individual to recognize all aspects of himself within his own consciousness. He has turned to the illusion that the mirror of life has presented. He becomes addicted to the compulsive pursuit of sexual conquest of others, trying to quench the thirst of his own soul for recognition of the whole person. Alas, he only sees what he seeks in others.

When one accepts a limited definition of himself, he experiences himself as such. In truth, we are more than any definition we have accepted of ourselves. The soul, knowing the truth, seeks to bring this awareness into consciousness. Everywhere one looks in the mirror of life, he sees only himself mirrored back in what he pursues. It is merely the outward illusion of what actually lies within him. Desire can be satisfied only when it is finally recognized in one's self. The tall dark man we all seek is ourself.

No one can judge promiscuous behavior for it is in truth only the reflection of the ego's desperate search for its own self fulfillment. However, each outward grasping is an act of self-denial, the acceptance of an illusion, until finally the true joy of life is squeezed out. Joy is the current on which the immune system runs. As there is less and less joy, then the immune system begins to weaken and the body is robbed of its ability to fight viruses and germs, and infection follows.

It has been popular for people both gay and straight to cry out against the outer circumstance of promiscuity as a curb to the spread of AIDS. It has been known from centuries of experience that morality cannot be legislated. The change can come only from within by the acceptance of the true self. Much of the legislation enacted concerning AIDS has taken the form of a judgment against homosexuality, the souls' true expression. That has only escalated the spread of AIDS, for judgment of homosexuality produces guilt. Guilt creates the lack of self love that is at the root of this disease.

Self-denial manifesting through our own sexuality is at the root of this problem. To understand we must look beyond the outward behavior to the inner cause, of which promiscuity is but a reflection. We must look at the limited meaning we have attached to what it means to be homosexual.

To be homosexual is more than a preference for certain sexual activities. The expression of our love for one another surely has dimensions beyond the mere physical act of sex. Have we so come to see ourselves in terms of our physical bodies that we see only the physical when we look at one another? Our modern obsession of body consciousness is reflecting back to us who we think we are. We are not just the sum totals of our body parts. We can not judge one another solely in terms of our pectoral muscles. We are more than our biceps. We are the light and the life behind our eyes.

Sexual union is more than the linking of two bodies. It is the joining of two hearts and minds as one. It is not solely recreational behavior, but is the extension of our intimacy with one another beyond the point where words can reach. When the creative energy of orgasm passes through our bodies, it is the loving connection in the heart that transforms it into a life-enhancing experience. This is the truest meaning of safe sex.

This cruel epidemic, which has taken so many of those we love, is in truth an opportunity. It is an opportunity to learn the greatest truth of all. It is the truth about ourselves. The liberation we experienced in the early seventies that allowed us to express our sexuality has now become a limitation. We have allowed these limited understandings to become the defining element of our lives. This is not the truth. They are a few small aspects of the glorious whole that we are. We must learn the truth about ourselves and then we will be able to see it in our brothers and sisters.

Sexual preference is not the defining factor of any life, straight or gay. Spirit cannot be limited by sexual roles. The sex act is much more than the joining of two physical bodies. It is an experience of moving beyond the body into a realization of our oneness in spirit.

Our attitudes toward sex have been very casual, but sexual energy is never casual. It is the same creative energy that brought us forth into being as divine ideas in the mind of God. It is this same energy, transformed through the loving human heart that empowers the creations of our own minds. We must expand to understand ourselves as whole lest we empower fragmentation and death. We must accept this and move beyond our use of such limiting definitions of selfhood.

It is time to move beyond our self-imposed isolation as a sexual minority. It is this isolation that creates the separation we experience from ourselves and society as a whole. When we reject the limited definition we have accepted of ourselves, then the outer barriers of societal discrimination keeping us apart will dissolve as if by magic. We cannot expect to receive from others what we have not dared to give ourselves. When we learn this then we as whole people will take our place proudly in the society of which we are such an important part. Our rights as homosexuals will not come through a piece of legislation. It will come from within, through the authority of a power far greater than any governmental body man can create.

△ FOCUS

One of the ways in which the mind creates reality for itself is through its focus. When the mind is focused on a goal, be it career or otherwise, the goal is created by the power of focus. By focusing upon a desired result, the goal is brought forward from the world of possibility and is manifested as the reality that is experienced.

The strength of the intent or desire behind the focus will determine just how rapidly the desired goal is materialized. The degree to which fear is allowed to frustrate the individual in the steps needed to bring the goal about will determine the degree of success in realizing the goal. Underlying beliefs in opposition to the desired goal also serve to sabotage the result. The rule of consciousness is such that you get what you focus upon.

What we focus on is given energy by that focus. The universe of matter is at its essence energy. That energy is directed by the tool of thought. When we focus our thoughts in a specific direction, we empower the object of our focus. The things which we cease to direct our thoughts toward begin to wither from the lack of energy directed at them. They cease to become a reality for us.

We are the creators of our personal reality and our focus is a tool by which we bring the desired reality into being. What we choose to give no thought to becomes of no effect for us. We always get what we focus on.

If we are to be healthy, it is health we must focus on. If it is disease we choose to focus on, that is what we will own. If a diseased person is to release the condition he finds himself in, then he must be able to turn his attention away from the condition.

It is not that he ignores the condition in which he finds himself but he accepts the condition only as an effect of his own consciousness. He then directs his attention, not towards the symptom, but inward towards consciousness, from which the symptom is but a message. When we receive a message, whether it is pleasing or not, we do not attack the messenger. Instead, we respond to the message. This is the correct course to take in dealing with illness.

By focusing on the disease condition, one continues to direct energy into the condition and maintain the condition. The patient must begin to shift the focus of his thoughts away from fighting the disease symptom toward the pursuit of wellness. The perception he holds must be shifted so he begins to see the condition in a different light. He must begin to see the opportunity that facing the situation affords, and begin to accept the message.

One of the biggest problems with AIDS, as it continues to increase in stature as a life-threatening epidemic, is that now there is a scientific medical blueprint for the disease which the patient can follow. He is told the syndrome of AIDS follows such and such a progression of opportunistic diseases, ever increasing in severity, finally culminating in death. He believes it is true. He believes science when it says he will die and rejects his own heart that speaks to him of hope. He expects his condition to worsen and it does. It is this blueprint upon which he turns the focus of his mind. It is this scenario that he accepts as truth.

Through the fear and belief the acceptance of this blueprint engenders, consciousness dutifully brings it into reality. What we accept as true, what we believe will happen, leads us to expect the result. That expectation goes forth as a magnet to attract the expected experience.

The gay community is gripped by the fear of AIDS. We fear we will be killed by this insidious virus. We expect it is inevitable. We accept that viruses are deadly carriers of disease from which we have no protection. We examine our bodies looking for spots we fear might be Kaposi Sarcoma. We feel our glands constantly, fearing they will be swollen. We turn the full focus of our minds on the accepted disease scenario in fear and expectation. Lo and behold, we find what we are looking for. We have accepted the condition by our focus, belief, expectation, and fear. The medical view of the body and the disease process is a limited and distorted one. It deals only with the physical, ignoring the deeper realities of being. In the case of AIDS, we must begin to accept a larger picture of what is really happening if we are to heal. We must begin to understand ourselves in terms that reach beyond the biological.

When we accept the scientific and medical belief that our bodies are weak physical specimens, at the whim of every passing germ or virus, and we carefully examine ourselves expecting to find the condition we fear, we create that very condition. You always get what you focus on.

True healing comes as an end result of our focus on finding our own wholeness. When we open our mind to our spiritual source and turn our focus on the task of reconnecting with that source, then we have begun to use the focus of our mind in a truly constructive way. This focus will bring into reality a dimension of power beyond what we have ever imagined for ourselves - the power of the God within. This power, unimpeded by the altered ego, transcends the action of any germ or virus.

It is not that we should not deal with our illness in physical terms but we should begin to nurture our bodies. We must stop attacking our symptoms. As we begin to give loving acceptance to both ourselves and our symptoms for their message to us, then we can release our experience in disease.

To activate the healing process there needs to be a shift in the focus of the afflicted. Focus gives power to the object of its intent. Dwelling on the illness strengthens its grip upon us. With a new understanding of the mental process involved in the initiation of the disease , we can now begin to look away from the present experience of disease. We can look inward toward the beliefs held in our own consciousness that limit us in any way.

We should not ignore our symptoms. Instead of struggling against them, however, we should realize that they are but the effect of an inner cause. We must focus on exploration of the contents of our own consciousness and the discovery of our true self, buried beneath limiting manmade structural concepts.

When one is willing to surrender his own limited concepts of self and search in honesty for the truth of his being, he will always find it. It has always been who he is, only hidden under layers of rigid beliefs to the contrary. This search for self will lead to the joyous discoveries of limitlessness that will begin to produce the uplifting emotions in the body necessary to restore health. The glands of the endocrine system await the emotional commands of true self love and discovery. These emotional charges flowing out of unlimitedness will stimulate the hormonal flow necessary to restore immune function in the body.

To alleviate the condition of AIDS, or any other disease condition, it is necessary to realize the true nature of the disease process. It stems from beliefs held in consciousness which are then translated through the emotional body by the mechanism of the endocrine glands into degrees of immunity in the physical body.

With AIDS we are dealing with the total collapse of the immune function brought about by a total dysfunction of the thymus gland. The thymus glands is where the T-cells that are destroyed by AIDS are brought to maturity. This gland is the physical correlate of the heart chakra and is activated by issues dealing with the giving and receiving of love.

To restore its function we must examine our attitudes toward ourself and our fellow man. We need to look at the fears we have around these issues. Fear is the lack of love. By the holding of unfounded fear we shut down the functioning of this center.

By our beliefs we experience our reality. We must become aware we are the creators of our experience, creating each moment and circumstance by our use of thought. We must find the beliefs we accept as fact about reality. One by one we must reject the beliefs in limitation which produce the fear by which we are imprisoned.

By the laws under which the mind operates, we empower that which we turn the focus of our mind upon. If we focus on resistance to our disease condition, as if it were a power unto itself, we empower the very symptoms we seek to alleviate. The disease is a symptom. The cause of the symptom lies in consciousness. It is there we must look for the solution.

We must focus on identifying and releasing the beliefs and structures we have accepted that give our power away to people and things outside ourselves. This release will always lead to the true joy of self in all its limitlessness. Joy is the current which will restore the immune system and deactivate the HIV virus, rendering it absolutely powerless against us.

There is no power outside of God. God is the reality within each one of us. The illusions of lack and limitation, disease, and suffering are empowered only by man's failure to realize his divine limitless self. The forces he fights against are shadows that he himself has created through belief. He has become lost in the dream of his own creation.

Man has but to awaken to his true nature to end his nightmares. When he does he will see the beauty of this life he has been given. He can then let go of every government, person, dogma, science, or belief that would tell him how he should live his life. He can then begin to follow the prompting of his own heart. Those promptings seek to lead him to the peace he searches for. Health and joy are found in self and its pure expression. When the focus of our mind is turned within, the illusions of mankind fall away.

So it is with AIDS. Seek first to discover the truth about yourself and all its glory, for there lies the answer. Do not resist the apparent symptoms of disease. Disease itself is but a reflection of limitations held in consciousness. Instead, seek to nurture the body and self. Remove the veils of limited understanding from your mind and the effect of illness will fall away. Do not be afraid.

Someone once said "There is nothing to fear but fear itself".

That is a great truth. You are in control of your life. It is your creation. Become aware of how you have created it and change it if you will. No one can do it for you and nothing can keep you from it.

You are the creator of your own life, a law unto yourself. Focus on your limitless self and by that focus, all the illusions you have empowered against yourself will wither from the loss of your energy. Only what is real will remain and that will be a joyful, healthy, and prosperous you.

WELLNESS PROCESS

I have tried to lay a groundwork so we may begin to look at ourselves in larger terms. Most of us have lived our lives as if asleep, unconsciously accepting the illusions we have created. We have lost the knowledge that we are the source from which our experiences emerge. In the realms of thought and feeling we exist in our truest sense.

Now with AIDS we are faced with a grave crisis which defies a medical cure. If there is to be a healing, it demands we look inwardly at our own thoughts and feelings. We must search for the ways we have contributed to this outer effect called AIDS. If we can enlarge our perspective of who we are we will be able to see the opportunity this condition offers to each one of us. It is a chance to know the truth about ourselves. This truth is one of limitless joy and health.

We each are the creators of our own life. We have the power to create for ourselves anything that can be imagined. Science is just now beginning to recognize the potential of the mind. This potential is far greater than science has imagined.

Through thought all that exists is created. Matter is the manifestation of thought expressed at its lowest frequency. Mind over matter is not some far out theory. Mind is the ruler of this physical reality and all other realities existing beyond our present perceptions.

Here in the physical world we come to learn of our true power in a medium where thought is slowed to its densest state, matter. If it were not slowed down, we would destroy ourselves in an instant by our fear. Instead through the psychological mechanism of time, our thoughts slowly emerge in linear fashion as the reality of our lives. In the game of life we face our own self-doubts so we can move beyond them into the creative role in the universe we all will someday assume.

Through our beliefs we have structured the reality we experience. Our beliefs give birth to the emotions we feel. They reach out into dimensions beyond this one, riding on electrical currents, and act as magnets, attracting back to us circumstances which confirm to us what we believe is fact. We then experience these beliefs as reality. Our reality is not set in concrete, however. It grows out of our beliefs about ourselves and our relationship to our environment, within the framework of our physical existence.

At the root of our human experiences of illness and lack lies a faulty belief about who we really are. From this one false belief, all of the distortions of what is true occur. We distort a reality of abundance and joy into the illusions of illness and lack through the misperceptions flowing out of our acceptance of an incorrect identity.

Out of our limiting beliefs we have created the negative emotions we experience. This negativity manifests in our bodies as disease and limitation. These are the outward physical products of our interior mental world. It is this interior world we must examine and change. We must turn inward to find our eternal reality from which the physical self emerges.

The history of the world is one long dark tale of war, famine, disease, and pestilence because man has not accepted his role as the creator of his circumstance. Millenniums of fighting against outer circumstance have produced very little in the way of peace and abundance. And little will emerge until man awakens to the role he himself is playing in creating his world.

Man has for too long thought of himself in physical terms, only. He will be forced to look inward if he is to find the solutions to the seemingly insurmountable problems he now faces. Like the dreaming man, experiencing the terrible nightmare of his subconscious creation, in reality he is safe in bed. So too physical man must awaken from the reincarnational dream of physical existence to find the limitless self that exists beyond this realm of illusion.

When one takes responsibility for the creation of his experience, he can begin to restore the current of joy on which the immune system runs. Out of the limitlessness we are in spirit flows a feeling of joy. This joy is responsible for the hormonal secretions creating healthy bodily functions. We must accept a new vision of ourselves as whole. Then we can begin the process of becoming more than we have dared dream. But we must first look at the beliefs we have accepted and rid ourselves of the ones serving to separate us from an experience of total freedom.

Disease is a reflection in the body of misaligned thinking. It is a physical expression of a false belief. To fight its symptoms is to shoot the messenger for the message it would bring. It is to succumb to the illusion. Its message is about the thoughts we hold about ourselves, from which the condition has its source. With AIDS we must focus on changing our mind if we are to see results.

The emotional states we experience, be they joy or frustration, flow out of beliefs. Every emotion we feel is caused by a belief held in consciousness. The negativity we feel is created by limiting beliefs we have accepted. These negative conditions separate us from the power of our true self and create the disease conditions in our body through the hormonal secretions of the endocrine system. By recognizing these beliefs one can begin to remove them and change the reality. These are only thoughts about reality and thoughts can be changed.

Begin to use the mirror that life presents you to examine things about yourself. When you look at others, what do you see? Beauty? Fear? Pain? You are looking at yourself. Use that knowledge to find yourself.

EXERCISES TO ASSIST YOU IN RELEASING AIDS

▲ Make a list of all the things that you believe to be true about yourself and the world around you. List all things the church, science, your parents, and your peers have told you. Examine the beliefs in vogue in the society in which you live.

▲ Now examine those beliefs in the light of your new identity as an unlimited being. How have you sold yourself short?

▲ Feel the emotion that flows from each belief. Notice when you feel less than joyful. Now you can see what thought in consciousness is blocking you from your unlimited experience.

▲ Recognize that you have created the condition. Through taking responsibility for our own life, we begin to empower ourselves. If this disease condition is our own creation, then we can choose to recreate it in another way. By not accepting responsibility we give power away to the condition.

▲ Recognize what you have created is an illusion of limitation. In truth you are whole. Your focus on the symptoms gives power to the illusion. The outer condition of disease is but the reflection of an inner cause. It is the result of one's misaligned thinking. Look within at the judgments held in consciousness.

▲ Remind yourself this is an opportunity to change. Love yourself and your condition for the opportunity it brings. You are not being punished for anything. Rather, you have created an experience that reflects your erroneous thoughts. You can choose to perceive the experience as a lesson and use it to correct your perceptions. In meditation ask what the message is for you.

▲ Replace the illusion with affirmations stating the truth. The truth is, your experience is but the result of distorted perceptions. Of itself it has no real power. Create an affirmation stating your own power. It will allow you to see through the delusion.

▲ Visualize how it would be to be well and healthy. Stay focused on ways to create health. The symptoms are but the message. To focus on the illness is to be deceived by the illusion. Focus and act upon ways that allow health to manifest. Explore ways to build a healthy immune system.

LOVING ACCEPTANCE

This last 25 years of the 20th century is indeed an exciting time in which to live. We approach not only the close of the 20th century, but the close of a millennium and the end of the Piscean Age. The twilight before the dawning of the age of Aquarius is the time of which sages of old and many ancient religious traditions have spoken of as the last days. All of us to some extent are aware of the scenarios of impending gloom and doom of which these traditions speak. Yet none of them need ever be.

The future can never be predicted with certainty. It is formed anew by decisions made in every present moment. These prophesies are merely probable futures we are creating for ourselves by our unconscious use of thought at this moment. These scenarios are pictures of the future we are creating with our consciousness of fear, lack, and separation. And yet they can be changed in any given moment by loving acceptance for all things. We are not locked into these disaster scenarios by some sadistic punishing God. We are ourselves the creators of these realities, with the ability to choose the future we will experience.

On every level, everyone on this planet is being brought to a point where they as individuals are being asked to look at the areas of their lives that are not in alignment with love. These areas are contributing to the mass realities of chaos and confusion being experienced on a global level. By facing up to self, we as individuals are casting our ballots for the scenarios we would see realized on the earth plane.

We have reached a point in the evolution of the planet and human consciousness upon it where our technological progress has so outstripped our spiritual understanding. In essence we are children playing with loaded guns. This lack of spiritual understanding has brought us to a point globally where our survival as a species, indeed the very survival of the planet itself, has been called into question. And yet survival is imminent. It is not within our abilities to stand against the surging tide of spiritual evolution.

In the body, when a cell or group of cells begins to act in a manner that is not conducive to the overall health of the body, but acts in a manner which is harmful to the organism as a whole, we experience this as disease, even cancer. At this point, the immune system of the body is called into action. The cellular activity is corrected or the misaligned cells are cleared from the system and health is restored.

Our physical bodies are a microcosm for the planetary body, the earth upon which we live. We as humans are as cells in that body. Through our misaligned thinking we have come to see ourselves as having interests separate from the interest of the species as a whole. We have become as cancerous cells on the body of the earth. We have exploited each other and the body of the planet to such an extent that on a massive scale, the earth's ecological system has been severely damaged. It has been strained to the point where it may soon no longer support life as we now know it. The earth must soon muster all the force within her to affect the healing that must come. One means of achieving this healing is the scenario of massive earth shifts and destruction, foretold for so long.

Consider AIDS as an aspect of global evolution; a mechanism through which the earth is affecting healing. It is one form in which the entire globe must confront the issues of love and respect for all life that is necessary for life on this planet to continue. As persons with AIDS must confront their own issues of self-love and respect for life in order to heal, so too must each one of us face these issues in our own way.

The lack of love for ourselves and one another is the soil in which this dis-ease grows. We, as a whole race of people, must look at how this illness, affecting only a part of humanity, is a creation and reflection of our global selves. AIDS reflects back to each one of us our inhumanity to one another. It provides the mirror through which we may see the end result of the disenfranchisement of any group of people.

AIDS does not exist as a punishment of any group, no matter how self-righteous some of us may feel and no matter how we try to place the blame outside of ourselves. AIDS mirrors to each and every one of us our part in the mass reality we all have had a hand in creating. This experience will not leave us until we all become a part of its solution. This is the gift of AIDS. When this disease has run its course, we will emerge on the other side of this experience as a changed race of people, one that recognizes and practices the loving acceptance of all people.

If we choose to place blame on those who manifest this disease, to judge against them because we don't like their choice of who to love, then we will continue to add fuel to feed the fire of this plague. That fire will be fanned by the winds of hate until it consumes all who would make these judgments.

No amount of legislation or quarantining will make anyone safe from this lesson. The hateful outcry of those who would place blame, make self-righteous judgments, and try to use this situation as a means to destroy those they hate and fear, will draw to them the very experience they fear. This is the creative power of thoughts projected through fear and hatred.

Potentially deadly viruses lie latent in every body alive on this planet. They are not necessarily passed along in the manner our sciences would have us believe. Viruses contribute to the overall health of every living thing on this planet and are present at all times. They respond to the environment in which they find themselves. They are triggered into hostile behavior by our own consciousness of fear and hatred. If we would end this disease then we must first deal with our attitudes.

Those who would protect themselves by hurting others will manifest disease for themselves if they continue to propagate hate. Disease is the natural result of a mind out of alignment with love. Exposure to an infected person is not necessary for illness to occur.

Homosexuality is not the issue here. At issue are the judgments we as society have made against one another. We have created an environment in which self-esteem has become impossible for some in this society. We must look at our judgments of one another if we are to find a cure.

When we choose to face this disease in loving acceptance for the messages it would bring us, then we will release this experience called AIDS. It brings a message of love and acceptance to every person on this planet. When this lesson is finally learned, the experience of AIDS will no longer be necessary.

Love is the cure for AIDS. Loving acceptance creates self-esteem. In turn, it is reflected out into our experience as behavior which is life enhancing, not death creating. The judgments we make against one another must end. These judgments are the breeding ground of AIDS. They must be replaced by loving acceptance. This is the true meaning of the last judgment.

Just as AIDS is a condition in man where the ability of the body to resist disease is impaired until death is the inevitable result, so too is the planetary body of the earth experiencing AIDS. Through lack of love and respect for all life we have plundered and polluted the soil and seas and atmosphere of this planet until it too is loosing its ability to sustain life.

The same denials and judgments in operation in the individual, leading to the AIDS condition, are also in operation on a global level. Just as an individual poisons his own body with drugs and self abuse, so too, as an entire race, are we doing the same to our planet.

On the eastern seaboard of the United States large number of dolphins and whales have washed ashore with wasted bodies, killed by a bacteria that not so long ago was not harmful to them. They suffer from an AIDS like condition. We express surprise and dismay at their death and demand an explanation. Yet daily we continue to dump toxic waste, sewage, and garbage into the rivers and sea, refusing to recognize the cause.

We have leveled our oxygen producing forests to such an extent the atmosphere no longer has the ability to replenish itself. We have destroyed our source of life-giving oxygen upon which we depend for breath. By our lack of knowledge of the interdependence and oneness of all life, we are in essence committing suicide as a species. Yet consistently we make choices based on superficial issues of greed.

Denial of this sort lies at the heart of AIDS, both individual and planetary. Until we choose to learn the lessons it presents, the problem will continue to grow. The simple fact is this planet can no longer support the level of destructive unconscious behavior we have been responsible for in the past. It has begun an unstoppable process necessary to bring about planetary healing. On an individual and planetary scale, we are facing the result of our misaligned thinking. It will move us into a greater alignment with life. No one will escape this tide of change. It is the coming of Christ-consciousness.

Those of us who are unable at this time to make the choice of loving acceptance necessary for the healing of the planet are being asked to leave. We are making our exits through AIDS, and war, and all manner of ways this technological society affords us. In dying some are able to achieve a healing. Death is not necessarily the failure we judge it to be for life is ongoing and eternal. These healings into death contribute to the lifting of the consciousness of the planet. Those who are healed in death will incarnate once again into the Aquarian Age on earth.

Several spiritual sources indicate that those unwilling to choose love over fear may not have an opportunity to return again to this planet. The spiritual body of the earth as a whole is evolving beyond a consciousness of fear. The vibration of fear will no longer match the new planetary vibration of love, and reincarnation for some will be rendered impossible.

This does not mean those who cannot return will be cast out into eternal damnation. Rather, the choice of returning to this planet will be rendered impossible. There are, however, many other planets in this vast universe available and able to support a continuation of karmic reincarnational learning. To these planets will those souls go, to continue the inevitable process by which each individual comes to choose love over fear.

It is not obligatory we choose love at this time. God's gift of free will allows us to choose in our own time, whenever that may be. The future of earth will be one of love and cooperation. Processes are increasingly being put into operation to bring about the necessary growth in human understanding. These processes begin with each one of us on the individual level. All change must begin with the individual. We decry our ability to affect policy on a global scale, but we fail to recognize that change begins with self. Then it ripples out from us, touching those with whose lives we come in contact, changing them and initiating a chain of events larger than we are ever aware of. And as each one of us becomes healed, so too is the planet healed. One day soon it will be reflected back to us in the new mass reality of love we will have created.

Love is the power that heals all things. We first learn to love and accept ourselves and then it spills over into our experience with one another. In the sharing of love comes the healing this planet so desperately cries for. Our resistances to love have created the conditions we find on earth today. By facing our resistance and releasing judgments the healing we seek will be allowed.

RECOMMENDED READING MATERIAL
Prepared by Wil Garcia and George Melton

AIDS and the Healer Within
Nick Bamforth/Amethyst Books

**The AIDS Book:
Creating A Positive Approach**
Louise L. Hay/Hay House

**AIDS: Passageway to
Transformation**
Carolyn Myss/Stillpoint Publishing

A Course in Miracles
Foundation for Inner Peace

Creative Visualization
Shakti Gawain/Whatever Publishing

Emmanuel's Book
Pat Rodegast & Judith Stanton
Friend's Press

Getting Well Again
Simonton & Simonton/Bantam Books

Heal Your Body
Louise L. Hay/Hay House

**The Healer Within - The New
Medicine of Mind & Body**
Steven Locke, MD & Douglas
Colligan/E. P. Dutton

Healing AIDS Naturally
Laurence E. Badgley, MD
Human Energy Press

Healing From Within
Dennis T. Jaffe/Simon & Schuster

The Healing Power Within
Ann Wigmore/Avery Publishing

**I'm Looking For Mr. Right, But
I'll Settle For Mr. Right Away**
Gregory Flood/Brob House Books

Life After Life
Raymond Moody/Walker & Co

Living With AIDS: Reaching Out
Tom O'Connor/Crowin Press

Living With Joy
Sanaya Roman/H. J. Kramer

Love, Medicine and Miracles
Bernie Siegel, MD/Harper & Row

The Nature of Personal Reality
Jane Roberts/Prentice-Hall

**Personal Power Through
Awareness**
Sanaya Roman/H. J. Kramer

**Psychoimmunity and the
Healing Process**
Jason Serinus/Celestial Arts

Reflections on the Path
Herbert Puryear/A.R.E. Press

Roger's Recovery From AIDS
Robert Owen/Davar

**The Secret of Instantaneous
Healing**
Harry Douglas Smith
Parker Publishing

Sex and the Spiritual Path
Herbert Puryear/A.R.E. Press

You Can Have It All
Arnold M. Patent
Celebration Publishing

You Can Heal Your Life
Louise L. Hay/Hay House

**AIDS Survivors Literature
(Catalogue)**
Project Survival, San Francisco, CA

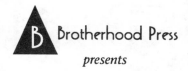

Brotherhood Press

presents

A MESSAGE OF INSPIRATION
Audio cassettes by Wil Garcia and George Melton

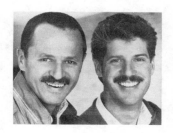

#101 – S.H.A.R.E. PEOPLE ARE HEALING FROM AIDS:
Live recording of a seminar on healing AIDS in which Wil & George
share their personal healing experiences. 90 minute cassette.

#102 – CONVERSATIONS WITH WIL & GEORGE:
Interview format in which Wil & George answer questions about AIDS
and the principles of self-healing. 90 minute cassette.

Produced and distributed by Brotherhood Press
279 S. Beverly Drive, Ste 185, Beverly Hills, CA 90212
For information or to book Wil and George for a seminar
call (213) 395-5667

ORDER FORM (Check or money order only)

Name _____

Address _____

City _____ State _____ Zip_____

Please send:	Qty	Price	Total
101 - S.H.A.R.E.		$10.00	
102 - CONVERSATIONS		$10.00	
201 - BEYOND AIDS (book)		$10.00	
California residents add 6.5% tax			
Shipping $1.50 (.75 each add. item)			
Total Enclosed			

Mail to Brotherhood Press, 279 S. Beverly Drive, Ste 185, Beverly Hills, CA 90212